Vegan Cook book

100 Simple Vegan Recipes for Beginners

Clark Johnson

Wait! Before You Begin... Are You a Vegan Looking to Lose A Few Pounds and Get in Shape?

If you answered YES then you are not alone. It is no secret that almost everyone wants to get in shape, build muscle, and look great. Unfortunately, most of us have no idea how to do it or where to even start! Yes- dieting and quick trips to the gym can work; but doing it wrong can lead to frustration and failure.

If you were hoping to find fitness tips tailor-made for your vegan lifestyle- then you've found the right place! Right now, you can get full **FREE access to 2 VEGAN FITNESS AND LIFESTYLE GUIDES.** These two reports are filled to the brim with crucial vegan fitness tips, hacks, and secrets! Become an instant vegan fitness pro after reading these **FREE GUIDES!**

Download 2 Of the Best Beginner Vegan Fitness and Health Guides to Help You Get in Shape Fast 100% FREE!

Vegan Healthy Lifestyle Hacks and Tricks
Beginner's Guide to Plant-Based Fitness

CLICK HERE FOR INSTANT ACCESS
http://bit.ly/2vy3zFs

Contents

Introduction

In recent years, the concept of a Vegan diet has quickly catapulted itself onto the main stage. Gaining massive popularity from nutritionists, dieticians, and regular people alike. This is all mainly due to the massive amount of positive effects that it gives the human body.

Individuals who are looking for an alternative to today's unhealthy diets are altering their lifestyle into a more "Vegan" path to stay fit and healthy in the long run.

Properly planned whole food vegan diets have been proven to reverse the effects of disease and help those trying to lose weight. Additionally, one of the main reasons for many switching to a vegan diet is that if planned properly, it can actually cost much less than any other diet.

As an added benefit, various other environmental and ethical issues are also at play here, which is helping Veganism gain traction with mainstream audiences.

In fact, recent studies and statistics show that almost 7.3 million Americans are considered to be Vegetarians and more than 1 million of them are pure Vegans.

On top of that, 22.8 million Americans are also supposedly following a diet that is simply a modified vegetarian routine.

If you have picked up or downloaded this book, then I am sure you are also inclined in following the same vegan path that many others have followed as well.

If that is the case, then I assure you that you going to the find the information and recipes in this book to be extremely helpful.

Before allowing you to jump into the recipes, let's start with the basics first!

What does a Vegan Diet mean?

Generally speaking, a vegan diet is a type of diet where a follower tries to exclude any and all form of produce that are even vaguely linked to animals. This means that produces such as meat, eggs, milk, cheese etc. are completely off the table.

A person who follows a vegan diet not only does so for the sake of staying healthy. In fact, the vegan lifestyle is often considered to be a revolution against animal cruelty and exploitation and a push for smarter environmental practices.

The people who follow a vegan diet will be filling up their plate with healthy greens and other fruits and vegetables.

One of the gray areas many people have is the difference between veganism and vegetarianism.

As mentioned before, individuals who follow a vegan diet completely restrict themselves from having any kind of animal/dairy products or anything that is even remotely related to animals.

On the other hand, vegetarians allow a degree of freedom in this matter by allowing animal derived products such as milk or eggs into their diets.

Just to make thing clear, the recipes in this book are completely targeted towards veganism.

Different types of Vegan Diets

That being said, you should keep in mind that there are actually plenty of different types of Vegan diets.

This allows people with different preferences the opportunity to tailor their vegan diet according to their requirements and desire.

While there are even more than the ones mentioned below, these are the more famous ones:

- **Whole food Vegan Diet:** This diet is by far the healthiest one to follow, it emphasizes eating different kinds of whole plant foods such as nuts, seeds, legumes, fruits, whole grains etc.
- **Raw-Food Vegan Diet:** This diet is composed of nuts, raw fruits, plant foods, vegetables, seeds that are cooked under a temperature of 118-degree Fahrenheit.
- **80/10/10:** This unique diet encourages an individual to rely on fat rich plants such as avocados and nuts and focuses more on raw fruits and tender greens. This diet is also known as "Fruitarian diet"
- **The Starch Solution:** This is similar to the aforementioned Fruitarian diet with the exception that it focuses on cooked starches such as rice, potatoes and corn instead of raw fruits.
- **Raw Till 4:** This is a low-fat diet that is a variation of the fruitarian and Starch Solution diet. In this diet, Raw fruits are consumed up until 4 PM, after which, the individual has the option to cook a nice plant based meal to end the day with.
- **Junk Food Vegan Diet:** This diet relies largely on mock meats and vegan compliant cheese, desserts and fries. Not to mention, other heavily processed vegan produces as well!

Despite the different between the types, the main aim should always be to eliminate meat from your diet and go for healthy greens instead.

General guidelines for the diet

If you are ever in a situation where you are confused as to what to eat, you can simply follow these guidelines to start your journey and say farewell to an unhealthy lifestyle.

- Try to eat at least five portions of veggies and fruits with loads of varieties each day.
- Make sure to keep your base meals revolved around rice, bread, potatoes, pasta and other starchy carbs.
- Go for dairy alternatives such as soya drinks and almond milk, coconut milk, etc.
- Try to pack some nuts and beans to ensure that you are supplied with protein.
- If using oil and spreads, make sure to go for unsaturated ones and in small portions.
- Make sure to keep yourself packed with lots of fluid, preferably 6-8 cups of water per day.

Allowed Foods

Here is a brief outline of the different types of foods that you are allowed to gobble up!

- **Tofu, Seitan and Tempeh:** These are excellent providers of protein and are great alternatives to fish, poultry and meat.
- **Legumes:** These include beans, peas and lentils, which are also great sources of many essential nutrients and beneficial plant compounds.
- **Nuts and Nut Butters:** Go for pure unroasted and unblanched ones as they are packed with selenium, zinc, fiber, iron etc.
- **Seeds:** Flaxseed, hemp and chia are good choices when it comes to seeds as they are packed with a good dose of omega-3 fatty acids and protein.
- **Algae:** Chlorella and Spirulina are amazing sources of protein and can be thrown into just about any meal.
- **Calcium Fortified Plant Milks And Yogurts:** These are excellent alternatives for a vegan to meet their daily recommended dietary calcium intake.
- **Nutritional Yeast:** This is yet another way of easily obtaining a large amount of protein from Vegan meals. Make sure to go for the ones that are labeled "Vitamin B12" fortified for maximum benefit.
- **Sprouted and Fermented Plant Foods:** Produces such as tempeh, natto, miso, pickles, kombucha and Kimchi fall under this category and they offer a good amount of vitamin K2 and probiotics.
- **Whole Grain Cereals and Pseudocereals:** These are good providers of complex carbs, iron and Vitamin B.

- **Vegetables and Fruits:** These should make up the bulk of your diet. They are amazing sources of nutrients. Leafy greens such as bok Choy, kale, mustard greens and even spinach are jam packed with calcium and iron.

Restricted Foods

These are the products you need to avoid on a vegan diet.

- **Meat:** Lamb, beef, veal, pork, chicken, wild meat, goose, turkey, quail, duck etc.
- **Fish and Seafood:** All types of sea food are restricted including squid, shrimp, anchovies, calamari, crab etc.
- **Eggs:** Any kind of eggs, including ostrich, quail, chicken, and fish are off the table.
- **Dairy:** Ice Cream, cheese, cream, milk, butter is restricted.
- **Animal Based Produces and Ingredients:** Such as whey, lactose, casein, egg white albumen, carmine, gelatin etc. are to be avoided.
- **Bee Products:** Such as royal jelly, pollen, honey etc. are to be avoided as well.

If you are new to the vegan diet and think you can't do it after reading that list, do not worry. The advantages of being a vegan more than make up for the sacrifices that are made, plus you will find out that transitioning is not as hard as it seems.

Amazing advantages of being a Vegan

- Protection from various chronic diseases such as Type 2 Diabetes
- Greatly reduce the possibility of you suffering from Cardiovascular diseases or Ischemic heart diseases
- Relieve your stress and keep you free from hypertension
- Lower the possibility of you suffering from stroke
- Helps prevent obesity
- Protect you against various cancers, including colon and prostate
- Increase the health of your bones preventing arthritis
- Increase your kidney functionality
- Helps prevent the development of Alzheimer's

And those are just the tip of the ice berg!

Some risks to keep in mind

Being a vegan requires that you have your house stocked with healthy fruits and vegetables constantly. However, it should be noted that there are a few nutrients you will need to specifically seek out since we are unable to get all desired nutrients from plants.

Therefore, it is highly recommended that you prepare a well-defined vegan plan before going into the diet, otherwise your body might suffer from certain vitamin and mineral deficiencies.

Since Vegans tend to replace all, if not most processed foods with plant based alternatives, they are a larger risk of suffering from Vitamin B12, Vitamin 2, Omega 3, Iron, Iodine, Zinc and Calcium deficiencies.

Therefore, a proper diet is a must. So, make sure to keep the following points in mind.

- Make sure to included foods that are fortified with calcium, vitamin B12 and Vitamin D on your plate. Examples include, fortified almond, rice milk, soy, orange juice, collard greens, turnip, bok choy, dried figs etc.
- Try to ferment sprouts and cook your food in order to enhance absorption of zinc and iron
- Make sure to use iron cast pots and pans while cooking and avoid drinking coffee or tea with iron rich foods
- A little bit of iodized salt or seaweed will help maintain appropriate iodine levels
- For long chain Omega-3's, go for chia, flax seeds, soybeans, hemp etc.

Vegans are also allowed to take supplements as well to make up for their deficiencies. Sometimes it's tough for an individual to properly follow all of the rules.

The below supplements should be kept in mind in order to make sure that you are eating a proper vegan diet.

- **Vitamin B12:** Try to take supplements that contain B12 in cyanocobalamin form for maximum effectiveness.
- **Vitamin D:** Go for D2 or Vegan D3 that are manufactured by Viridian or Nordic Naturals.
- **EPA and DHA:** Take from algae oil, also able to get some from chia seeds
- **Iron:** Should only be ingested through means of supplements should you face deficiency. Otherwise, avoid taking extra Iron.
- **Iodine:** Either take supplements or add 1/2 a teaspoon of iodize salt to your daily diet.
- **Calcium:** Take tablets of 500mg or less daily.
- **Zinc:** Take in forms of Zinc Citrate or Zinc Gluconate. Make sure that you are not to take these while taking Calcium supplements.

Fantastic tips to encourage weight loss through Veganism

By now you have already understood that veganism won't directly help you trim down your weight, rather it will indirectly help you to burn excess fats.

Aside from eating fiber rich veggies and fruits, the following tips will greatly increase the effectiveness of your diet in terms of losing weight!

- When undergoing a vegan transition, initially it might be really hard to resist the temptation of meat. Therefore, it is of utmost importance that you create a very strong mindset where you accept the fact that you are not allowed to go for any meat, it's all mental. In short, you are to embrace the absence of meat. This will make your vegan journey easier.
- Don't increase your intake of desserts and breads just because they are "vegan compliant". Cut them down to one portion at least and especially avoid sodas!
- Try to go for high protein and low-fat smoothies to keep your muscles pumped instead of fruit juices. They will help absorb the essential nutrients faster. Just make sure to replace the base milk with non-dairy products such as unsweetened soy milk.
- Make sure to cut back on your sugar intake as it will make it much harder for you to lose weight.
- Don't hesitate to go for green leafy vegetables such as bok Choy, collard greens, mustard etc. They will provide you with a good dose of calcium, which will make your weight loss effort more efficient.

- Keep in mind that simply eating veggies won't trim down your weight if you just sit around all day! Try to get some aerobic exercise in order to maximize your effort. Even a 30 minutes treadmill walk will do! Just make sure to do a warm up session of 15 minutes before starting your exercise.

Vegetables and Fruits for Weight Loss

These are some of the best fruits and veggies that you would want to keep an eye out for to encourage your weight loss.

- Broccoli
- Green/Red Peppers
- Spinach
- Pickles
- Potatoes
- Onions
- Black Beans
- Avocado
- Oats
- Blueberries
- Pears
- Grapefruit
- Kidney Beans
- Almonds
- Lentils
- Banana

Chapter 1
Breakfast Recipes

Super Vegan Oatmeal Smoothie

Prepping time: 10 minutes
Cooking time: 0 minutes
For 2 servings

Ingredients:

- 1 cup of almond milk or coconut milk
- ½ a cup of rolled oats
- 14 frozen strawberries
- 1 banana broken up into chunks
- 1/2 a cup of blueberries
- 1 and a 1/2 teaspoons of agave nectar
- 1/2 teaspoon of vanilla extract

Preparation:

- Open up your blender and add all of the listed ingredients together
- Blend the whole mixture until smooth
- Chill and serve!

Nutrition Values

- Calories: 205
- Fat: 2.9g
- Carbohydrates: 42g
- Protein: 4.6g

Luxurious Lemon Poppy Seed Scones

Prepping time: 10 minutes
Cooking time: 15 minutes
For 12 servings

Ingredients:

- 2 cups of all-purpose flour
- 3/4 cup of white sugar
- 4 teaspoon of baking powder
- 1/2 teaspoon of salt
- 3/4 cup of margarine
- 1 zested and juiced lemon (lime also works)
- 2 tablespoons of poppy seeds
- 1/2 a cup of soy milk
- 1/2 a cup of water

Preparation:

- Pre-heat your oven to a temperature of 400-degree Fahrenheit
- Take a baking sheet and grease it up well
- Take a large sized bowl and stir in the flour, baking powder, sugar and salt
- Toss in the margarine into the mixture until it shows a consistency of large grains of sand
- Make sure to continue rubbing the margarine as you cut it into the flour with your hand
- Stir in poppy seeds, lemon juice and lemon zest once you have received your desired consistency
- Take another bowl and add soy milk and water
- Gradually stir this mixture into the bowl with dry ingredients until the batter it moist, yet thick similar to biscuit dough

- Spoon 1/4 cup sized portions of the dough into your greased baking sheet and keep them 3 inches apart
- Bake in your oven for about 15 minutes
- Serve!

Nutrition Values

- Calories: 240
- Fat: 12g
- Carbohydrates: 30g
- Protein: 3g

Simple Scrambled Tofu

Prepping time: 10 minutes
Cooking time: 15 minutes
For 4 servings

Ingredients:

- 1 tablespoon of olive oil
- 1 bunch of chopped up green onion
- 1 chopped up garlic clove
- 1 can of peeled and diced tomatoes
- 1 pack of firm silken tofu drained and mashed up
- Ground turmeric for taste
- Salt as needed
- Pepper as needed

Preparation:

- Take a medium sized skillet and place it over medium heat
- Heat it up and drizzle in the olive oil
- Add the onions and sauté them until tender
- Add the tomatoes and mashed tofu while stirring
- Season with some pepper, salt, turmeric, and garlic
- Lower down the heat and allow it to simmer until thoroughly heated
- Serve and enjoy!

Nutrition Values

- Calories: 200
- Fat: 11g
- Carbohydrates: 9.7g
- Protein: 14g

Homestyle Fried Potatoes

Prepping time: 10 minutes
Cooking time: 15 minutes
For 6 servings

Ingredients:

- 1/3 cup of shortening
- 6 large sized peeled and cubed potatoes
- 1 teaspoon of salt
- 1 teaspoon of ground black pepper
- 1/2 a teaspoon of garlic powder
- 1/2 a teaspoon of paprika

Preparation:

- Take a large sized iron skillet and add shortening
- Heat it up over medium heat
- Add potatoes and cook them by stirring until they show a fine golden-brown texture
- Season them with pepper, salt, paprika and garlic
- Serve hot!

Nutrition Values

- Calories: 326
- Fat: 11g
- Carbohydrates: 52g
- Protein: 5g

Silky Smooth Strawberry Oatmeal Smoothie

Prepping time: 10 minutes
Cooking time: 15 minutes
For 2 servings

Ingredients:

- 1 cup of almond milk
- 1/2 a cup of rolled oats
- 16 frozen strawberries
- 1 cut up mango
- 1/4 cup of chia seeds
- 1 banana broken up into chunks
- 1 and a 1/2 teaspoons of agave nectar
- 1/2 a teaspoon of vanilla extract

Preparation:

- Open up your blender and add all of the listed ingredients together except for the vanilla extract
- Blend the whole mixture until smooth
- Add vanilla extract and sugar if you want a sweeter taste
- Chill and serve!

Nutrition Values

- Calories: 236
- Fat: 3.7g
- Carbohydrates: 44g
- Protein: 7.6g

Healthy Pistou

Prepping time: 10 minutes
Cooking time: 25 minutes
For 4 servings

Ingredients:

- 1 tablespoon of rapeseed oil
- 3 finely sliced leeks
- 1 large sized finely diced courgette
- 1 L of boiling vegetable stock
- 400g of can of cannellini
- 200g of chopped green beans
- 4 chopped tomatoes
- 2 finely chopped garlic cloves
- Small pinch of basil
- 40g of fresh vegan cheese (optional)

Preparation:

- Take a large pan, add oil and heat it up
- Add leeks and the courgette then fry for 5 minutes
- Pour stock and add 4 quarters of cannellini and green beans
- Add half of your tomatoes and lower down the heat, allow it to simmer for 8 minutes
- Add the mixture to your food processor alongside beans and tomatoes
- Mix well and stir in vegan cheese (optional)
- Stir the soup into the frying pan and cook for 1 minute. Serve hot!

Nutrition Values

- Protein: 12g
- Carbs: 19g
- Fats: 12g
- Calories: 210

Hardy Steel Cut Oats and Quinoa

Prepping time: 5 minutes
Cooking time: 20 minutes
For 4 servings

Ingredients:

- 3 cups of water
- 1/2 a cup of quinoa
- 1/2 a cup of steel-cut oats
- 2 tablespoons of almond meal
- 2 tablespoon of flaxseed meal
- 1/2 tablespoon of ground cinnamon

Preparation:

- Take a saucepan and add in water
- Bring the water to a boil
- Add oats and quinoa
- Simmer the mixture well, making sure to keep stirring it from time to time until the water has been fully absorbed, should not take more than 20 minutes
- Stir in the almond and flaxseed meal into your quinoa
- Pour the mixture into a glass container
- Garnish with cinnamon
- Allow it to cool for about 15 minutes
- Serve or transfer it to your fridge and serve later!

Nutrition Values

- Calories: 180
- Fat: 4.7g
- Carbohydrates: 30g
- Protein: 8g

Perfect Vegan Pancakes

Prepping time: 5 minutes
Cooking time: 10 minutes
For 3 servings

Ingredients:

- 1 and a 1/4 cup of all-purpose flour
- 1 and 1/2 tablespoons of white sugar
- 2 teaspoons of baking powder
- 1/2 a teaspoon of salt
- 1 and a 1/4 cup of water
- 1 tablespoon of oil

Preparation:

- Take a large sized bowl and pour in flour, baking powder, and sugar
- Next, take a small bowl and whisk the water and oil together
- Make a well at the center of your bowl from step 1 and pour the water and oil mix in
- Stir until finely blended (should show a lumpy texture)
- Take a lightly oiled up griddle and place it over medium-high heat
- Drop the batter into the griddle (large spoonfuls) and cook them until bubbles form and the edges become dry
- Flip and cook until nicely browned
- Keep repeating until all of the batter has been used up!

Nutrition Values

- Calories: 250
- Fat: 5.1g
- Carbohydrates: 52g
- Protein: 5.3g

Sweet and Simple Baked Apples

Prepping time: 5 minutes
Cooking time: 20 minutes
For 1 servings

Ingredients:

- A couple of your favorite apples (Fuji works well)
- Raisins as needed
- Cinnamon as needed
- Maple Syrup as needed

Preparation:

- Pre-heat your oven to 350 degrees Fahrenheit
- Core the apples nicely
- Stuff the apples with raisin, maple syrup and cinnamon
- Add them to your prepared oven and bake for 20 minutes
- Serve!

Nutrition Values

- Calories: 98
- Fat: 0.27g
- Carbohydrates: 42g
- Protein: 0.43g

Personal Kale and Banana Smoothie

Prepping time: 5 minutes
Cooking time: 0 minutes
For 1 servings

Ingredients:

- 1 piece of banana
- 2 cups of chopped kale
- 1/2 a cup of light unsweetened soy milk
- 1 and a 1/2 tablespoons of chia seed
- 1 teaspoon of maple syrup

Preparation:

- Open up your blender and add all of the listed ingredients together
- Blend the whole mixture until smooth
- Chill and serve!

Nutrition Values

- Calories: 320
- Fat: 7.3g
- Carbohydrates: 56g
- Protein: 12g

Easy to Make Carrot Balls

Prepping time: 10 minutes
Cooking time: 0 minutes
For 10 servings

Ingredients:

- 6 pieces of pitted Mejdool dates
- 1 finely grated carrot
- 1/3 cup of raw walnuts
- 1/4 cup of unsweetened finely shredded coconut
- 1 teaspoon of nutmeg
- 1/8 teaspoon of sea salt

Preparation:

- Take a food processor and add in dates, 1/4 cup of grated carrots, coconut, salt and nutmeg
- Mix the whole mixture and puree it
- Add the rest of the walnuts and 1/4 cup of carrots. Pulse the mixture well until it has a clunky texture
- Using your hand, form 10 small sized balls roll them up in your coconut
- Add some carrots as topping and chill them
- Serve!

Nutrition Values

- Calories: 326
- Fat: 16g
- Carbohydrates: 42g
- Protein: 3g

Filling Oat Bran Cereal

Prepping time: 5 minutes
Cooking time: 5 minutes
For 1 servings

Ingredients:

- 1 cup of water
- 1/4of a teaspoon of ground cinnamon
- 6 dried and pitted prunes (chopped up)
- 1/4 cup of oat bran

Preparation:

- Take a saucepan and place it over medium heat
- Add water, cinnamon, prunes and bring the whole mixture to a boil
- Stir in oat bran and boil for about 2 minutes
- Serve!

Nutrition Values

- Calories: 140
- Fat: 1.9g
- Carbohydrates: 42g
- Protein: 5.2g

Easy Cornmeal Slices

Prepping time: 5 minutes
Cooking time: 5 minutes
For 1 servings

Ingredients:

- 1 and a 1/4 cup of cornmeal
- 2 cups of water
- 1/2 a teaspoon of salt

Preparation:

- Take a saucepan and place it over medium heat
- Add cornmeal, salt and water and cook the mixture for 5-7 minutes until a thick mixture has formed
- Pour the mixture into a loaf pan and allow it to chill
- Cut it into slices and remove them from the pan
- Fry them over medium-high heat in hot oil until both sides are browned
- Serve and enjoy!

Nutrition Values

- Calories: 90
- Fat: 0.4g
- Carbohydrates: 17g
- Protein: 1.6g

Guilt Free Vegan Waffles

Prepping time: 5 minutes
Cooking time: 5 minutes
For 6 servings

Ingredients:

- 1/3 cup of water
- 2 tablespoons of flax seed meal
- 1 cup of rolled oats
- 1 and 3/4 cups of almond milk
- 1/2 a cup of all-purpose flour
- 1/2 a cup of whole wheat flour
- 2 tablespoons of canola oil
- 4 teaspoons of baking powder
- 1 teaspoon of vanilla extract
- 1 tablespoon of agave nectar
- 1/2 a teaspoon of salt

Preparation:

- Pre-heat your waffle iron according to the instructions (of the waffle iron)
- Take a bowl and stir in water and flax seed meal
- Take your blender and blend the oats until they show a flour like consistency
- Add the flax seed mixture, flour, almond milk, whole wheat flour, canola oil, vanilla extract, baking powder, agave nectar and salt to your oats
- Blend the whole batter well until mixed
- Ladle 1/2 a cup of the batter into your waffle iron
- Cook until a golden crisp texture shows (for about 5 minutes)

- Serve and enjoy!

Nutrition Values

- Calories: 240
- Fat: 8g
- Carbohydrates: 34g
- Protein: 7g

Wild Samoan Panikeke

Prepping time: 10 minutes
Cooking time: 30 minutes
For 12 servings

Ingredients:

- 3 and 1/3 cups of all-purpose flour
- 1 and a 1/3 cup of white sugar
- 2 teaspoons of baking powder
- 2 ripe mashed bananas
- 1 tablespoon of vanilla extract
- 1 and a 1/2 cup of water
- 5 cups of vegetable oil

Preparation:

- Take a large sized bowl and add flour, baking powder and sugar
- Thoroughly mix them
- Stir in bananas, water and vanilla extract and keep mixing it until the dough is sticky
- Take a large sized saucepan and add oil
- Place it over high heat and heat up the oil to 350-degree Fahrenheit (make sure that oil is 3 inches deep)
- Scoop up 1/4 cup of the batter with a large sized spoon and use another spoon to push the panikeke off into the oil
- Fry in small batches of 4-5 pieces until they float to the top and show a nice golden-brown color (should take around 3 minutes)
- Flip them carefully and fry the other side
- Remove and drain them

- Serve!

Nutrition Values

- Calories: 345
- Fat: 11g
- Carbohydrates: 57g
- Protein: 5g

Delightful Millet Meal

Prepping time: 15 minutes
Cooking time: 75 minutes
For 4 servings

Ingredients:

- 1 cup of uncooked millet
- 1/2 a cup of soy milk powder
- 5cups of hot water
- 2/3 cups of chopped up dates
- 1/2 a cup of flaked coconut
- 1 teaspoon of vanilla extract

Preparation:

- Pre-heat your oven to 350 degrees Fahrenheit
- Take your 9x13 inch casserole pan out and add millet, hot water, soy milk, coconut, chopped dates, vanilla
- Bake in your oven for about 30 minutes and remove
- Give it a stir
- Return to your oven and bake for another 30 minutes
- Serve hot!

Nutrition Values

- Calories: 180
- Fat: 3.9g
- Carbohydrates: 32g
- Protein: 6.9g

Soulful Avocado Toast

Prepping time: 10 minutes
Cooking time: 0 minutes
For 4 servings

Ingredients:

- 4 slices of whole grain bread
- 1 halved and pitted avocado
- 1 tablespoon of chopped fresh parsley
- 1 and a 1/2 teaspoons of extra virgin olive oil
- 1/2 a teaspoon of salt
- 1/2 a teaspoon of ground black pepper
- 1/2 a teaspoon of onion powder
- 1/2 a teaspoon of garlic powder

Preparation:

- Toast your bread in your toaster well
- Scoop avocado into a bowl
- Add parsley, olive oil, salt, onion powder, pepper, garlic powder and mash everything together using a potato masher
- Spread the avocado mix into your piece of toast
- Serve!

Nutrition Values

- Calories: 170
- Fat: 10g
- Carbohydrates: 16g
- Protein: 7g

Avocado Toast Bites (Party Favorite!)

Prepping time: 10 minutes
Cooking time: 3 minutes
For 2 servings

Ingredients:

- 1 slice up of toasted whole wheat bread
- 1/2 of a sliced avocado
- Flaky sea salt or pink Himalayan salt
- Freshly cracked black pepper
- Good quality olive oil
- Crushed up red pepper flakes

Preparation:

- Cut the avocado slices properly and spread them on top of your bread in a fan shape
- Using a fork, mash the avocado slices carefully
- Sprinkle a bit of black pepper and salt
- Drizzle olive oil and garnish with some pepper flakes
- Enjoy!

Nutrition Values

- Protein: 7g
- Carbs: 28g
- Fats: 15g
- Calories: 250

Smooth Almond Berry Smoothie

Prepping time: 10 minutes
Cooking time: 0 minutes
For 1 servings

Ingredients:

- 1 cup of frozen blueberries
- 1 cup of frozen strawberries
- 1 cut up banana
- 1/2 a cup of almond milk
- 1 tablespoon of almond butter
- Water as needed

Preparation:

- Add all of the listed ingredients into your blender and blend until a smooth mixture appears
- Add as much water as you need to thin the smoothie
- Chill and serve!

Nutrition Values

- Calories: 315
- Fat: 10g
- Carbohydrates: 53g
- Protein: 5.5g

Hearty Nuts and Granola Mix

Prepping time: 10 minutes
Cooking time: 35 minutes
For 6 servings

Ingredients:

- 2 cups of rolled oats
- 1/2 a cup of spelt flour
- 1/3 a cup of packed brown sugar
- 1 teaspoon of ground cinnamon
- 1 teaspoon of ground ginger
- 3 tablespoons of canola oil
- 1/4a cup of unsweetened applesauce
- 3 tablespoons of maple syrup
- 1/4a cup of diced dried apricots
- 1/4a cup of chopped pecans
- 3 tablespoons of chia seeds (ground)

Preparation:

- Pre-heat your oven to a temperature of 300 degrees Fahrenheit
- Take a baking sheet and line it up with parchment paper
- Toss rolled oats, spelt flour, cinnamon, brown sugar, ginger, apple sauce, canola oil, maple syrup, dried apricots, ground chia seed and pecans to a bowl
- Mix well
- Spread the whole mixture on your lined baking sheet
- Bake for about 20 minutes
- Stir the granola carefully
- Bake for another 15 minutes until the mixture is dry

- Allow it to cool down and serve and enjoy!

Nutrition Values

- Calories: 385
- Fat: 15g
- Carbohydrates: 57g
- Protein: 7g

Chapter 2
Lunch Recipes

Delightful Peanut and Edamame Noodle Salad

Prepping time: 10 minutes
Cooking time: 2 minutes
For 4 servings

Ingredients:

- 3 bags of 8-ounce Shirataki noodles, drained and rinsed
- 2 cups of frozen corn
- 1/2 a cup of organic peanut butter
- 1/2 a cup of rice vinegar
- 1 tablespoon of Sriracha hot sauce
- 1/4 cup of water
- 1/2 a teaspoon of salt
- 3 cups of shredded carrots
- 16 ounce of halved grape tomatoes
- 1 medium sized quartered and sliced Granny Smith apples
- 1/2 a cup of freshly chopped cilantro

Preparation:

- Take a large sized saucepot and add water
- Place it over high heat and allow it to boil
- Add Shirataki noodles, corn and Edamame and boil for 2 minutes
- Rinse and drain them well
- Take a large sized bowl and add peanut butter, Sriracha hot sauce, salt, water and rice vinegar

- Add shredded carrots, apples, tomatoes, noodle mix and cilantro
- Toss everything well
- Garnish with some additional sriracha
- Enjoy!

Nutrition Values

- Calories: 455
- Fat: 4g
- Carbohydrates: 50g
- Protein: 25g

Vegan Linguine with Wild Mushrooms

Prepping time: 10 minutes
Cooking time: 5 minutes
For 6 servings

Ingredients:

- 1 pound of linguine
- 5 tablespoons of olive oil
- 12 ounces of mixed mushrooms thinly sliced up
- 3 and 1/2 finely chopped garlic cloves
- 1/4 cup of nutritional yeast
- 2 thinly sliced green onions

Preparation:

- Cook the linguine as properly instructed on the pack
- Once done, drain the pot but make sure to reserve 3/4 cup of pasta cooking water
- Return the drained linguine to your pot
- Take a 12-inch skillet and add oil, place it over medium-high heat
- Add garlic and mushroom and sauté them for 5 minutes
- Transfer them to the pot with your drained linguine
- Add nutritional yeast, cooking water, 3/4 teaspoon of coarsely ground pepper and 1/2 a teaspoon of salt
- Toss everything well
- Garnish with some green onion
- Enjoy!

Nutrition Values

- Calories: 430

- Fat: 15g
- Carbohydrates: 62g
- Protein: 15g

Crispy Potatoes with Amazing Vegan Nachos

Prepping time: 15 minutes
Cooking time: 30 minutes
For 4 servings

Ingredients:

- 2 pounds of mixed and halved baby potatoes
- 2 tablespoons of canola oil
- 1 cup of raw, unsalted cashews soaked overnight
- 2 tablespoons of lemon juice
- 1/2 a teaspoon of chili powder
- 1/2 a teaspoon of sweet paprika
- 1/3 a teaspoon of garlic powder
- 1 teaspoon of Coarse sea salt
- 1/4 cup of nutritional yeast
- 1/2 a cup of jalapeno chili, chopped and seeded

Preparation:

- Pre-heat your oven to a temperature of 450 degrees Fahrenheit
- Take a bowl and add potatoes, 1/2 a teaspoon of salt, oil and 1/4 teaspoon of pepper
- Take a rimmed baking sheet and spread the potatoes evenly
- Roast for 30 minutes
- Take a blender and add lemon juice, cashews, chili powder, paprika cumin, garlic powder, sea salt, yeast and jalapeno
- Add 1 cup of water
- Puree the mixture well
- Transfer the mixture to a 2-quart saucepan and simmer the mixture for 5 minutes over low heat

- Transfer the vegan sauce to a bowl
- Serve with the roasted potatoes!

Nutrition Values

- Calories: 390
- Fat: 18g
- Carbohydrates: 48g
- Protein: 10

Classic Baked Mexican Beans Dish

Prepping time: 5 minutes
Cooking time: 15 minutes
For 4 servings

Ingredients:

- 2 large sized Desiree Potatoes
- 14 ounce of Mexican Beans (caned)
- 4 cups of water
- 1.7 ounce of vegan butter
- 1.7 ounce of vegan cheese
- Parsley as needed

Preparation:

- Wash the potatoes thoroughly
- Cut the top part of the potatoes with X's and gently place the potatoes in a microwave proof dish
- Microwave on LOW for 15 minutes until they are soft and have split at the X point
- Remove and split with a fork
- Top the potatoes with Mexican Beans, cheese, parsley and butter
- Enjoy!

Nutrition Values

- Calories: 130
- Fat: 7g
- Carbohydrates: 6g
- Protein: 10g

Onion and Beet Avocado Salad

Prepping time: 10 minutes
Cooking time: 20 minutes
For 4 servings

Ingredients:

- 3 chopped up green onions
- 1/4 cup of lemon juice
- 2 tablespoons of olive oil
- 1 small shallots finely chopped up
- 5 ounce of baby kale
- 8 ounces of precooked, chopped up beets
- 2 thinly sliced ripe avocados
- 2 sheets of matzo crushed up into bite sized portions

Preparation:

- Take a large sized rimmed baking sheet
- Spray the onions with a bit of cooking spray and sprinkle 1/2 a teaspoon of salt onto them
- Add the onions to the baking sheet and bake for 15 minutes at 400-degree Fahrenheit
- Take a bowl and whisk in lemon juice, shallot, olive oil, 1/4 teaspoon of salt and 1/4 teaspoon of pepper
- Add half of the beets and baby kale and toss everything well
- Divide the mix onto your serving plates
- Top them up with matzo, avocados, onions (all thinly sliced up)
- Serve and enjoy!

Nutrition Values

- Calories: 330
- Fat: 26g
- Carbohydrates: 32g
- Protein: 7g

Homestyle Minestrone Soup

Prepping time: 10 minutes
Cooking time: 35 minutes
For 4 servings

Ingredients:

- 2 tablespoons of olive oil
- 3 chopped up medium sized carrots
- 1 thinly sliced medium leek
- 3 chopped up large red potatoes
- 8 cups of vegetable broth
- 1 bunch of sliced asparagus
- 1 can of 15 ounces drained and rinsed navy beans
- 2 tablespoons of chopped fresh chopped dill

Preparation:

- Take a 8 quart saucepot and add 2 tablespoons of olive oil and place it over medium heat
- Add carrots, leek and 1/4 teaspoon of salt
- Cook for 7 minutes, making sure to keep stirring it well
- Add chopped up red potatoes, vegetable broth
- Partially cover and allow the mixture to boil
- Lower down the heat to simmer and cook for 25 minutes
- Add asparagus and simmer for 3 minutes
- Stir in the navy beans, 1/4 teaspoon of salt, fresh dill and 1/2 a teaspoon of pepper
- Enjoy!

Nutrition Values

- Calories: 320
- Fat: 7g
- Carbohydrates: 60g
- Protein: 7g

Finely Spiced and Breaded Tofu

Prepping time: 15 minutes
Cooking time: 15 minutes
For 4 servings

Ingredients:

- 1 pack of 16-ounce extra firm and drained tofu
- 2 cups of vegetable broth
- 2 tablespoons of vegetable oil
- 1/2 a cup of all-purpose flour
- 3 tablespoons of nutritional yeast
- 1 teaspoon of salt
- 1/2 a teaspoon of freshly ground black pepper
- 1/2 a teaspoon of sage
- 1/2 a teaspoon of cayenne pepper

Preparation:

- Cut up the pressed tofu into 1/2-inch-thick slices
- Cut them again into 1/2-inch-wide sticks
- Add the tofu in a bowl and pour the broth on top of them
- Allow them to soak on the side
- Take another bowl and add in flour, salt, yeast, sage, pepper, and cayenne, then mix them together
- Take a large sized skillet and place it over medium high heat
- Add oil
- Remove the tofu sticks from the broth and squeeze the liquid
- Roll the sticks into the breading
- Place the coated tofu in your skillet and fry them till they are brown on all sides
- Enjoy!

Nutrition Values

- Calories: 330
- Fat: 7g
- Carbohydrates: 62g
- Protein: 7g

Healthy Orzo and Mushroom Soup

Prepping time: 5 minutes
Cooking time: 25 minutes
For 6 servings

Ingredients:

- 1 tablespoon of extra virgin olive oil
- 1/4 teaspoon of kosher salt
- 1 cup of chopped celery
- 1/2 cup of garlic
- 8 cups of vegetable broth
- 3 cups of broccoli
- 3 cups of sliced spinach
- 1 cup of sliced mushrooms
- 1 cup of orzo

Preparation:

- Take a 8 quart saucepot and add olive oil and place it over medium heat
- Add celery, salt, garlic and shallots
- Cook for 8 minutes until golden
- Add broccoli, broth and simmer them on high heat
- Lower down the heat to medium low and simmer for 15 minutes
- Add mushrooms, spinach, orzo and simmer for another 8-10 minutes
- Remove the heat and carefully stir in basil pesto
- Stir and enjoy!

Nutrition Values

- Calories: 350
- Fat: 7g
- Carbohydrates: 62g
- Protein: 7g

Mean Green Smoothie Drink

Prepping time: 10 minutes
Cooking time: 0 minutes
For 2 servings

Ingredients:

- 2 cups of coconut water
- 3 ounces of spinach
- 1 tablespoon of peanut butter
- 3 small sized bananas
- 1 teaspoon of vanilla essence
- 1 tablespoon of hemp seeds
- 1 tablespoon of chia seeds

Preparation:

- Carefully place all of the ingredients into a blender and blend them well
- Chill and serve!

Nutrition Values

- Calories: 289
- Fat: 6g
- Carbohydrates: 55g
- Protein: 6g

Grilled Up Asparagus Tacos

Prepping time: 15 minutes
Cooking time: 5 minutes
For 4 servings

Ingredients:

- 2 tablespoons of canola oil
- 4 crushed garlic cloves
- 1 tablespoon of ground chipotle chile
- 1 teaspoon of ground kosher salt
- 9 ounce of shiitake mushrooms
- 1 bunch of trimmed green onion
- 8 warmed corn tortillas
- 1 cup of homemade guacamole
- Lime wedges as needed
- Cilantro sprigs
- Hot sauce for serving

Preparation:

- Set your grill to medium
- Take a large sized baking dish and add oil, salt, garlic and chipotle
- Add asparagus, green onions, shiitakes and toss them well
- Grill the asparagus until they are tender for about 5-6 minutes
- Grill the shiitake and green onions for 4-5 minutes until they are slightly charred
- Transfer the grilled veggies to a cutting board
- Cut the asparagus and green onions to 2-inch length
- Slice up the shiitake

- Serve with guacamole, lime wedges, corn tortillas, hot sauce and cilantro
- Enjoy!

Nutrition Values

- Calories: 350
- Fat: 25g
- Carbohydrates: 36g
- Protein: 7g

Morocco's Special Couscous Stew

Prepping time: 15 minutes
Cooking time: 10 minutes
For 4 servings

Ingredients:

- 1 and 1/2 cups of vegetable broth
- 1 cup of couscous
- 1 teaspoon of olive oil
- 1 zucchini chopped up
- 1 cup of shredded carrot
- 1/4 cup of golden raisins
- 4 green onions
- 1 teaspoon of ground cumin
- 1 can of stewed tomatoes
- 1 can of chickpeas
- 2 teaspoons of Sriracha hot sauce

Preparation:

- Take a 1-quart saucepan and add 1 cup of vegetable broth
- Bring it to a boil over high heat
- Stir in the couscous and allow it to stand for 5 minutes
- Take a 12-inch skillet and add olive oil over medium heat
- Add zucchini and cook for 6 minutes, stirring well
- Add shredded carrots, green onions, ground cumin, and golden raisins
- Cook for 2 minutes
- Stir in stewed tomatoes, Sriracha hot sauce, chickpeas and 1/2 a cup of vegetable broth
- Break up the tomatoes using a spoon

- Simmer for 6 minutes
- Enjoy!

Nutrition Values

- Calories: 190
- Fat: 8g
- Carbohydrates: 124g
- Protein: 34g

Simple Fresh Pea Soup

Prepping time: 5 minutes
Cooking time: 5 minutes
For 4 servings

Ingredients:

- 18 ounces of frozen baby peas
- 2 cups of vegetable stock
- 1 cup of coriander leaves finely chopped up
- 1 cup of finely chopped up mint leaves
- Sea salt as needed
- Freshly ground pepper as needed

Preparation:

- Take a medium sized pot and add vegetable stock
- Bring it to a boil
- Add frozen peas and cook them for 3 minutes
- Add chopped up fresh herbs and mix with a spoon until it is all nicely blended and smooth
- Season with salt and pepper
- Enjoy!

Nutrition Values

- Calories: 690
- Fat: 29g
- Carbohydrates: 74g
- Protein: 25g

Bulgur Pilaf and Garbanzos

Prepping time: 10 minutes
Cooking time: 20 minutes
For 4 servings

Ingredients:

- 1 cup of water
- 1 can of vegetable broth
- 1 cup of bulgur
- 1 tablespoon of olive oil
- 1 small sized onion
- 2 teaspoons of curry powder
- 1 clove of garlic
- 1 can of garbanzo beans
- 1/2 a cup of dried apricot
- 1/2 a teaspoon of salt
- 1/4 cup of fresh parsley leaves

Preparation:

- Take a 2-quartsaucepan out then ass water and 1 and a 1/4 cups of vegetable broth and bring it to a boil over high heat
- Stir in bulgur and bring it to a boil
- Lower down the heat to medium-low and simmer for 15 minutes (covered)
- Remove the saucepan from the heat and fluff up the bulgur with fork
- Take a bowl and place it over a 12-inch skillet and heat up oil over medium for 1 minute
- Add onions and cook for 10 minutes and keep stirring it well
- Stir in curry powder and garlic and cook for 1 minute

- Stir in garbanzo beans, salt, apricots and ½ a cup of broth
- Bring the mixture to a boil
- Remove the heat and stir in the bulgur and parsley
- Enjoy!

Nutrition Values

- Calories: 230
- Fat: 4g
- Carbohydrates: 35g
- Protein: 7g

Delicious Veggie and Red Lentil Soup

Prepping time: 10 minutes
Cooking time: 10 minutes
For 4 servings

Ingredients:

- 1 tablespoon of olive oil
- 5 medium sized carrots
- 2 cups of water
- 1 small sized onion
- 1 teaspoon of ground cumin
- 1 can of diced up tomatoes
- 1 can of vegetable broth
- 1 cup of dried red lentils
- 1/4 teaspoon of salt
- 1/8 teaspoon of ground black pepper
- 1 bag of baby spinach

Preparation:

- Take a 4-quart saucepan and add oil
- Heat it up over medium heat until hot
- Add the onion and carrots then cook them for 6-8 minutes
- Stir in cumin and cook for 1 minute
- Add broth, lentils, tomatoes, 2 cups of water, salt and pepper
- Cover it up and bring the heat to a boil
- Lower down the heat to a simmer and cook for 8-10 minutes until the lentils are soft
- Stir in spinach
- Enjoy!

Nutrition Values

- Calories: 510
- Fat: 39g
- Carbohydrates: 12g
- Protein: 15g

Veggie Lo Mein

Prepping time: 10 minutes
Cooking time: 10 minutes
For 4 servings

Ingredients:

- 1 pack of extra firm tofu
- 1 cup of water
- 1 package of linguine
- 1 tablespoon of olive oil
- 1 chopped up celery stick
- 1/2 a cup of chopped up garlic cloves
- 1 teaspoon of ground pepper
- 1 chopped up zucchini
- 3 chopped up carrots
- 1 tablespoon of soy sauce
- 1 teaspoon of cilantro

Preparation:

- Cut up the tofu into blocks and half them lengthwise
- Cut up each of the pieces into 1/2-inch-thick slices
- Add the slices in a single layer between paper towels and remove any moisture
- Take a 12-inch skillet and add 1-inch water
- Bring it to a boil
- Add linguine and cook as specified
- Drain the linguine and rinse them under cold water
- In the same skillet, add 1 tablespoon of oil over medium heat and heat it for 1 minute

- Add the tofu in a single layer and cook them for about 10 minutes until they are golden brown, transfer to a plate
- In the same skillet and 1 tablespoon of oil and heat over medium heat for 1 minute
- Add celery, garlic, pepper and cook for 2 minutes until they are crisp and tender
- Add zucchini and cook for 1-2 minutes until they are crispy
- Add carrots, tofu, soy sauce and noodles
- Cook for 2 minutes over high heat
- Remove the heat and stir in sesame oil, garnish with cilantro and enjoy!

Nutrition Values

- Calories: 130
- Fat: 10g
- Carbohydrates: 30g
- Protein: 9g

Corn Chowder for Two

Prepping time: 15 minutes
Cooking time: 15 minutes
For 2 servings

Ingredients

- 5 peeled and chopped potatoes
- 2 cups of frozen corn
- 3 minced garlic cloves
- 1 chopped red pepper
- 1 chopped yellow onion
- 2 teaspoons of paprika
- 2 cups of vegetable broth
- 1 can of light coconut milk
- Salt as needed
- Chopped up green onion and cilantro for garnish
- Red pepper

Preparation:

- Chop up the onion and mince the garlic
- Add them to your pot
- Chop up the potatoes and red pepper and keep them aside
- Sauté the ingredients in your pot and add 1/4 cup of broth
- Take a spatula or long wooden spoon and keep stirring the onion and garlic for 5 minutes while they are being sautéed
- Add the rest of the listed ingredients
- Lock up the lid and let it cook for 8 minutes
- Once done, let the pressure release naturally by slowly releasing the lid
- If you want your soup to be thicker, blend it a bit

- Serve it over some rice or with a garnish of green onion, cilantro, red pepper and corn

Nutrition Values

- Calories: 50
- Fat: 4.4g
- Carbohydrates: 3.1g
- Protein: 1g

Fresh Orange and Onion Salad

Prepping time: 15 minutes
Cooking time: 15 minutes
For 2 servings

Ingredients

- 5 large orange pieces
- 2 tablespoons of red wine vinegar
- 4 tablespoons of olive oil
- 1 teaspoon of dried oregano
- 1 red onion thinly sliced up
- 1 cup of olive oil
- 1/4 cup of chopped fresh chives
- Ground black pepper

Preparation:

- Peel the oranges and cut each one into 4-5 crosswise slices
- Transfer them onto a shallow serving dish
- Sprinkle vinegar, olive oil, and oregano
- Toss gently
- Allow it to refrigerate for 30 minutes
- Toss again
- Arrange the sliced-up onions and black olives on top
- Decorate
- Sprinkle some chives and grind a bit of fresh pepper
- Enjoy!

Nutrition Values

- Calories: 238
- Fat: 12g
- Carbohydrates: 25g
- Protein: 3g

Ultimate Fried Bread

Prepping time: 5 minutes
Cooking time: 15 minutes
For 2 servings

Ingredients

- 1 tablespoon of olive oil
- 2 cups of all-purpose flour
- 1 tablespoon of baking powder
- 1 teaspoon of salt
- ¾ cup of water

Preparation

- Take a large sized saucepan and heat up the oil at 350 degrees Fahrenheit
- Take a large bowl and add flour, salt, and baking powder
- Mix well
- Add water and keep mixing until you can turn it into a ball with a slightly sticky consistency (takes around 5 minutes)
- Tear off plum sized portions from the ball and flatten them into 1/2-inch disks
- Fry the pieces in the hot oil until both sides are browned, should not take more than 3 minutes
- Drain and enjoy!

Nutrition Values

- Calories: 355
- Fat: 8g
- Carbohydrates: 62g
- Protein: 9g

Supreme Mexican Guacamole

Prepping time: 5 minutes
Cooking time: 5 minutes
For 6 servings

Ingredients

- 1 large sized avocado
- 1/4a cup of finely chopped red onion
- 1 juiced lime
- 1 finely chopped sprig cilantro
- 1 pinch of salt

Preparation

- Halve up the avocado vertically and gently remove the pit
- Next, use a knife and cut vertically and then horizontally into the avocado
- Take a spoon and scoop out the cubed avocado pieces from the skin
- Place them in a small bowl
- Mash the avocado chunks
- Mix in the lime juice, salt, lime onion and cilantro
- Serve!

Nutrition Values

- Calories: 65
- Fat: 4.4g
- Carbohydrates: 3.1g
- Protein: 2g

Mango Tahini Smoothie

Prepping time: 10 minutes
Cooking time: 0 minutes
For 2 servings

Ingredients

- 2 cups of frozen mango chunks
- 1 cup of water or almond milk
- 2 tablespoons of tahini
- 2 tablespoon of lime juice

Preparation

- Take a blender and add mango, tahini, water, lime juice and blend everything well
- Serve chilled!

Nutrition Values

- Calories: 190
- Fat: 8g
- Carbohydrates: 28g
- Protein: 3g

Chapter 3
Dinner Recipes

Winter's Delightful Turmeric Soup (Stock Pot Recipe)

Prepping time: 5 minutes
Cooking time: 25 minutes
For 4 servings

Ingredients:

- 5 teaspoons of vegan stock
- 3 cups of chopped carrots
- 1/2 an inch nub of fresh ginger
- 1/2 a cup of walnuts
- 1 teaspoon of turmeric
- 1/2 a teaspoon of cumin
- 1/2 a teaspoon of cinnamon
- 1 teaspoon of garlic powder
- 1 teaspoon of lemon juice
- 1 teaspoon of chipotle paste

Preparation:

- Add the ingredients to your stock pot and allow it to simmer for about 25 minutes
- Blend the whole mixture in a blender and enjoy warm!

Nutrition Values

- Calories: 210
- Fat: 4g
- Carbohydrates: 40g
- Protein: 10g

Amazing Ginger Stir Fry and Veggies

Prepping time: 25 minutes
Cooking time: 15 minutes
For 6 servings

Ingredients:

- 1 tablespoon of cornstarch
- 1 crushed garlic clove
- 2 teaspoons of chopped and fresh ginger root
- 1/4 of a cup of vegetable oil
- 1 small head of broccoli florets
- 1/2 a cup of snow peas
- 3/4 of a cup of julienned carrots
- 1/2 a cup of halved green beans
- 2 tablespoons of soy sauce
- 1/2 a cup of chopped onion
- 1/2 a tablespoon of salt

Preparation:

- Take a large sized bowl and add cornstarch, 1 teaspoon of ginger, garlic, 2 tablespoon of vegetable oil and mix well until the cornstarch has fully dissolved
- Mix the broccoli, snow peas, green beans and carrots
- Toss well
- Take a large skillet and place it over medium heat
- Add 2 tablespoons of oil and heat it up
- Cook the veggies in the oil for 2 minutes, making sure to keep stirring it frequently
- Stir in soy sauce and water
- Mix in salt, onion and 1 teaspoon of ginger

- Cook until the veggies are tender and crisp
- Enjoy!

Nutrition Values

- Calories: 130
- Fat: 9.3g
- Carbohydrates: 8g
- Protein: 2.2g

Stir Fried Garbanzo Dish

Prepping time: 15 minutes
Cooking time: 30 minutes
For 6 servings

Ingredients:

- 2 tablespoons of olive oil
- 1 tablespoon of chopped fresh oregano
- 1 tablespoon of chopped fresh basil
- 1 crushed garlic clove
- Ground black pepper
- 1 can of garbanzo beans
- 1 large sized zucchini – chopped up
- 1/2 a cup of sliced mushrooms
- 1 tablespoon of chopped fresh cilantro
- 1 chopped tomato

Preparation:

- Take a large sized skillet and place it over medium heat
- Heat up the oil
- Stir in oregano, basil, garlic and pepper
- Add garbanzo beans and zucchini then stir well to coat the herbs with oil
- Cover it and cook for 10 minutes, making sure to keep stirring it from time to time
- Stir in cilantro and mushrooms then cook until they are tender
- Add chopped up tomato on top of the mixture
- Cover and allow the tomatoes to steam for a while
- Serve hot!

Nutrition Values

- Calories: 145
- Fat: 7g
- Carbohydrates: 19g
- Protein: 4g

Mixed Rice and Cuban Beans

Prepping time: 10 minutes
Cooking time: 50 minutes
For 6 servings

Ingredients:

- 1 tablespoon of olive oil
- 1 cup of chopped onion
- 1 chopped green bell pepper
- 1 clove of minced garlic
- 1 teaspoon of salt
- 4 tablespoons of tomato paste
- 1 can of kidney beans, drained liquid
- 1 cup of uncooked white rice

Preparation:

- Take a large sized saucepan and place it over medium heat
- Add oil and heat it up
- Add bell pepper, onion, and garlic thensauté them
- Next, add salt and tomato paste then cook on low heat for 2 minutes
- Stir in the rice and beans
- Pour the liquid from the beans into a large sized measuring cup and add additional water to reach about 2 and a 1/2 cup of volume
- Pour the mix onto the beans
- Cover and cook on low 45-50 minutes
- Serve and enjoy!

Nutrition Values

- Calories: 240
- Fat: 6g
- Carbohydrates: 45g
- Protein: 7g

Simplistic Masoor Daal of Calcutta

Prepping time: 5 minutes
Cooking time: 30 minutes
For 4 servings

Ingredients:

- 1 cup of red lentils
- 1 sliced up ginger nub sliced into 1-inch pieces and peeled
- 1/4 teaspoon of ground turmeric
- 1/2 a teaspoon of salt
- 1/2 a teaspoon of cayenne pepper
- 3 teaspoons of vegetable oil
- 4 teaspoons dried minced onion
- 1 teaspoon of cumin seeds

Preparation:

- Rinse lentils thoroughly and wash them
- Take a medium sized saucepan and add salt, ginger, turmeric, cayenne pepper
- Cover about 1 inch of water and bring it to a boil
- Skim any foam from the top
- Lower down the heat and allow it to simmer until the beans are soupy and soft
- Take a microwave safe dish and add oil, dried onion and cumin seeds
- Microwave for 45 seconds on HIGH
- Stir the mixture into the lentils
- Enjoy!

Nutrition Values

- Calories: 170
- Fat: 5g
- Carbohydrates: 25g
- Protein: 12g

Olive Oil and Basil Pasta

Prepping time: 15 minutes
Cooking time: 10 minutes
For 8 servings

Ingredients:

- 1 pack of farfalle pasta
- 2 roma tomatoes, seeded and diced up
- 3 tablespoons of olive oil
- 2 minced garlic cloves
- 1/2 a cup of fresh basil leaves cut up into thin strips
- Salt as needed
- Pepper as needed

Preparation:

- Take a large sized pot and add salted water
- Place it over high heat and bring it to a boil
- Cook the pasta for about 8-10 minutes until Al-Dente
- Take a large sized bowl and add pasta, olive oil, tomatoes, garlic and basil
- Season with pepper and salt
- Enjoy!

Nutrition Values

- Calories: 320
- Fat: 14g
- Carbohydrates: 42g
- Protein: 8g

Classic Vegetable Curry

Prepping time: 5 minutes
Cooking time: 40 minutes
For 5 servings

Ingredients:

- 1 tablespoon of olive oil
- 1 chopped onion
- 2 crushed garlic cloves
- 2 tablespoons of curry powder
- 2 tablespoon of tomato paste
- 1 can of diced tomatoes
- 1 cube of vegetable bouillon
- 1 pack of frozen mixed vegetables
- 2 cups of water
- Salt as needed
- Pepper as needed
- 2 tablespoons of chopped fresh cilantro

Preparation:

- Take a large sized saucepan and place it over medium-high heat
- Add oil and heat it up
- Saute onions and garlic until golden
- Stir in curry powder and tomato paste and cook them for about 2-3 minutes
- Stir in tomatoes, mixed vegetables, vegetable bouillon, salt, pepper and water into the pan
- Cook for another 30 minutes until the veggies are tender
- Sprinkle a bit of cilantro

- Enjoy!

Nutrition Values

- Calories: 90
- Fat: 3.5g
- Carbohydrates: 15g
- Protein: 3.5g

Worldly Aloo Matar

Prepping time: 15 minutes
Cooking time: 30 minutes
For 4 servings

Ingredients:

- 1/4 cup of vegetable oil
- 3 medium sized finely chopped onion
- 1 tablespoon of ginger garlic paste
- 1 bay leaf
- 4 large sized peeled and chopped up potatoes
- 1 cup of frozen peas
- 1/2 a cup of tomato puree
- 1 teaspoon of garam masala
- 1 and a 1/2 teaspoon of paprika
- 1 teaspoon of white sugar
- 1 teaspoon of salt
- 2 tablespoons of chopped cilantro

Preparation:

- Take a wok and place it over medium heat, add oil and heat it up
- Stir in onion, garlic paste, ginger and the bay leaf
- Cook until the onions are tender
- Mix in potatoes and peas
- Cover and cook the potatoes for 15 minutes until they are soft
- Stir in tomato puree, sugar, paprika, Garam masala, salt and sugar into the vegetable mix
- Keep cooking for 10 minutes

- Add cilantro and cook for another 2 minutes
- Enjoy!

Nutrition Values

- Calories: 473
- Fat: 14g
- Carbohydrates: 81g
- Protein: 10g

Greatest Bean Curry Ever

Prepping time: 15 minutes
Cooking time: 70 minutes
For 4 servings

Ingredients:

- 1 tablespoon of olive oil
- 1 large sized chopped onion
- 1/2 a cup of dry lentils
- 2 minced garlic cloves
- 4 tablespoons of curry powder
- 1 teaspoon of ground cumin
- 1 pinch of cayenne pepper
- 1 can of crushed tomato
- 1 can of garbanzo beans drained and rinsed
- 1 can of kidney beans drained and rinse
- 1/2 a cup of golden raisins
- Salt as needed
- Pepper as needed

Preparation:

- Take a large sized pot and add oil then place it on medium heat
- Add onion and cook them until tender
- Add lentils and garlic and season with curry powder, cayenne pepper and cumin
- Cook and stir for 2 minutes
- Stir in tomatoes, kidney beans, garbanzo beans, raisins
- Season with some pepper and salt

- Lower down the heat to low and simmer for about 60 minutes
- Keep stirring occasionally
- Once done, enjoy!

Nutrition Values

- Calories: 195
- Fat: 4.7g
- Carbohydrates: 30g
- Protein: 8.9g

Delicious Mushroom Kabobs

Prepping time: 30 minutes
Cooking time: 10 minutes
For 4 servings

Ingredients:

- 3 sliced fresh mushrooms
- 2 red bell peppers chopped up
- 1 green bell pepper cut up into 1-inch pieces
- 1/4 cup of olive oil
- 2 tablespoons of lemon juice
- 1 minced garlic clove
- 2 teaspoons of chopped fresh thyme
- 1 teaspoon of chopped fresh rosemary
- 1/4 teaspoon of salt
- 1/4 teaspoon of ground black pepper

Preparation:

- Pre-heat your grill to medium heat
- Thread the mushrooms and pepper alternatively into your skewers
- Take a small sized bowl and add olive oil, garlic, thyme, lemon juice, salt, pepper and rosemary
- Brush the mushroom and pepper with this mixture
- Brush up the grate with oil
- Place the kabobs on the grill
- Keep basting from time to time
- Cook for 4-6 minutes until the mushrooms are tender
- Enjoy!

Nutrition Values

- Calories: 145
- Fat: 12g
- Carbohydrates: 9g
- Protein: 2g

Green Curry Tofu

Prepping time: 20 minutes
Cooking time: 25 minutes
For 4 servings

Ingredients:

- 2 cups of water
- 1 cup of uncooked basmati rice rinsed and drained
- 3 tablespoons of sesame oil
- 1 pack of firm water packed tofu drained and cubed
- 1/4 teaspoon of salt
- 1 can of coconut milk (can also use almond or soy milk)
- 2 tablespoons of green curry paste

Preparation:

- Take a medium sized saucepan and add water
- Bring the water to a boil over high heat
- Lower the heat and simmer for 20 minutes
- Remove the heat and allow it to cool
- Take another medium saucepan and place it over medium heat
- Heat up the sesame oil
- Stir in tofu and fry for 20 minutes until they are evenly crisp and until they are lightly browned
- Season with some salt
- Take a final small sized saucepan and bring the coconut milk to a boil
- Mix in green curry paste
- Lower down the heat and simmer for 5 minutes
- Drizzle the mixture over tofu and rice

- Serve!

Nutrition Values

- Calories: 525
- Fat: 35g
- Carbohydrates: 40g
- Protein: 27g

Tropical Pineapple with Teriyaki Tofu

Prepping time: 10 minutes
Cooking time: 20 minutes
For 4 servings

Ingredients:

- 1 pack of firm tofu
- 1 cup of chopped fresh pineapple
- 2 cups of teriyaki sauce

Preparation:

- Cut up the tofu into bite sized portions and place it in a deep baking dish
- Add pineapple
- Pour teriyaki sauce and allow it to chill for 1 hour
- Pre-heat your oven to 350-degree Fahrenheit
- Bake in your oven for 20 minutes until it is hot and becomes bubbly
- Take it out and serve!

Nutrition Values

- Calories: 250
- Fat: 8g
- Carbohydrates: 30g
- Protein: 22g

Marinated Portobello Mushrooms

Prepping time: 10 minutes
Cooking time: 33 minutes
For 4 servings

Ingredients:

- 1/2 a cup of cooking wine
- 1 tablespoon of olive oil
- 2 tablespoons of soy sauce
- 2 tablespoons of balsamic vinegar
- 2 cloves of garlic minced up
- 2 large Portobello caps

Preparation:

- Pre-heat your oven to a temperature of 400-degree Fahrenheit
- Take a baking dish and add wine, olive oil, balsamic vinegar, soy sauce and garlic
- Add mushroom caps upside down into the prepared marinade and allow it to marinate for 15 minutes
- Cover up the dish and bake for 25 minutes
- Turn the mushrooms, and keep baking for 8 minutes
- Enjoy!

Nutrition Values

- Calories: 112
- Fat: 6g
- Carbohydrates: 4g
- Protein: 1.3g

Quinoa Chard Pilaf

Prepping time: 20 minutes
Cooking time: 20 minutes
For 8 servings

Ingredients:

- 1 tablespoon of olive oil
- 1 diced onion
- 3 minced garlic cloves
- 2 cups of uncooked rinsed quinoa
- 1 cup of canned lentils rinsed up
- 8 ounces of fresh mushrooms
- 1 quart of vegetable broth

Preparation:

- Take a large sized pot and place it over medium heat
- Heat up the oil
- Stir in the onion and garlic then sauté for 5 minutes until the onions are soft
- Mix in quinoa, mushrooms, lentils
- Pour the broth and cook while covered for 20 minutes
- Next, keep it covered but allow it to sit for 5 additional minutes
- Enjoy!

Nutrition Values

- Calories: 215
- Fat: 5g
- Carbohydrates: 36g
- Protein: 10g

Teriyaki Seasoned Stir Fried Zoodles

Prepping time: 10 minutes
Cooking time: 12 minutes
For 2 servings

Ingredients:

- 1 tablespoon of olive oil
- 1 tablespoon of teriyaki sauce
- 1 large sized thinly sliced carrot
- 1/2 of a large sized green bell pepper thinly sliced up
- 1/4 of a large sized yellow onion thinly sliced up
- 1 bok choy head
- 1 large sized zucchini cut up into long strands
- 1 teaspoon of garlic powder

Preparation:

- Take a large sized skillet and place it over medium heat
- Add olive oil and 1 tablespoon of teriyaki sauce then heat it up
- Add the carrot, onion and bell pepper then cook until the onions become translucent for (usually takes around 5 minutes)
- Stir in the bok choy, garlic powder, and zucchini
- Drizzle any remaining teriyaki sauce and cook for another 7 minutes, frequently stirring until the zucchini noodles are soft
- Enjoy!

Nutrition Values

- Calories: 155
- Fat: 7g
- Carbohydrates: 20g
- Protein: 6g

Perfect Pascal Pasta

Prepping time: 10 minutes
Cooking time: 15 minutes
For 4 servings

Ingredients:

- 4 tablespoons of olive oil
- 3 minced garlic cloves
- 1 chopped onion
- 4 roma tomatoes diced up
- 1/2 a teaspoon of dried oregano
- 1/2 a teaspoon of dried basil
- Salt as needed
- Pepper as needed
- 1 pound of angel hair pasta

Preparation:

- Take a medium sized skillet and place it over medium high heat
- Add in your olive oil and heat it up
- Sautéthe garlic in the skillet for 1-2 minutes
- Toss in the onions and cook for 2 minutes more
- Stir in tomatoes, salt, pepper, basil and lower down the heat to let it simmer
- Take a large sized pot and add salted water
- Bring it to a boil
- Add pasta and cook for 3-5 minutes until al dente
- Drain
- Toss the pasta around with the tomato mix
- Serve and enjoy!

Nutrition Values

- Calories: 450
- Fat: 20g
- Carbohydrates: 65g
- Protein: 14.3g

Very Creamy Avocado Pasta

Prepping time: 20 minutes
Cooking time: 10 minutes
For 4 servings

Ingredients:

- 1 avocado cut into chunks
- 1 handful of cherry tomatoes
- 1/3 a cup of water
- 1 small handful of fresh basil
- 1 handful of spinach
- 1/4 cup of nutritional yeast
- 1 handful of chopped mushrooms

Preparation:

- Cook your pasta until al dente
- Take a blender and add in avocado, nutritional yeast, water, and basil
- Blend them until it becomes a smooth and runny texture
- Transfer the sauce to a bowl and mix it with the pasta
- Serve and enjoy!

Nutrition Values

- Calories: 245
- Fat: 9g
- Carbohydrates: 17g
- Protein: 9g

Homestyle Black Eyed Peas Blend on Soft Tortillas

Prepping time: 10 minutes
Cooking time: 15 minutes
For 4 servings

Ingredients:

- 1 tablespoon of olive oil
- 1/2 a cup of finely chopped onion
- 1 can of black eyes peas
- 1 fresh jalapeno pepper chopped up
- 1/2 a cup of vegetable stock
- 1/2 a cup of freshly cut red bell peppers
- 1 clove of minced garlic
- 1 tablespoon of fresh lime juice
- Salt as needed
- Pepper as needed
- Salt as needed
- Pepper as needed
- 4 pieces of 12-inch tortillas

Preparation:

- Take a medium sized skillet and place it over medium heat then add olive oil
- Heat it up and add the onion, cook until tender
- Mix in black eyed peas, jalapeno, red bell peppers, vegetable stock, lime juice, and garlic
- Season with some salt and pepper
- Keep cooking until thoroughly heated
- Put the mixture onto your tortillas and serve!

Nutrition Values

- Calories: 465
- Fat: 13g
- Carbohydrates: 73g
- Protein: 14g

Classic Veggie Fajitas

Prepping time: 30 minutes
Cooking time: 20 minutes
For 4 servings

Ingredients:

- 2 teaspoons of olive oil
- 2 minced garlic cloves
- 2 sliced green bell peppers
- 2 sliced yellow bell pepper
- 1/2 of a sliced onion
- 1 cup of sliced mushrooms
- 3 chopped green onions
- Lemon pepper as needed
- 1 fresh jalapeno pepper (optional if you want more spice)

Preparation:

- Take a large sized frying pan and place it over medium heat
- Add olive oil then sautéthe garlic for 2 minutes
- Stir in the sliced yellow and green bell peppers
- Sauté for an additional 2 minutes
- Stir in the onion and jalapeno then sauté for another 2 minutes
- Finally add green onions and mushrooms to the pan
- Season with lemon pepper and stir
- Cover and cook until the veggies are tender
- Enjoy!

Nutrition Values

- Calories: 57
- Fat: 2g
- Carbohydrates: 8g
- Protein: 4g

Southern Style Fried Tempeh

Prepping time: 5 minutes
Cooking time: 5 minutes
For 4 servings

Ingredients:

- 2 garlic cloves
- Some hot sauce as needed
- 1 cup of water
- Salt as needed
- 1 pack of tempeh (8 ounce)
- 2 cups of vegetable oil

Preparation:

- Take a mixing bowl and add garlic
- Pour water and salt in the bowl and mix everything
- Slice up the tempeh into 1-inch-thickpieces and score both sides thoroughly
- Marinate the tempeh in the garlic/water salt mixture for about 20 minutes
- Pan fry the tempeh in a skillet with oil
- Make sure it is brown and crispy on all sides
- Enjoy!

Nutrition Values

- Calories: 215
- Fat: 15g
- Carbohydrates: 5.8g
- Protein: 12g

Chapter 4
Snack Recipes

Yummy Chocolate Cherry Bars

Prepping time: 15 minutes
Cooking time: 0 minutes
For 14 servings

Ingredients:

- 2 cups of oats
- 1/2 a cup of quinoa
- 1/3 a cup of chia seeds
- 1/4 a cup of sliced almonds
- 1/2 a cup of dried cherries
- 1/2 a cup of chopped dark chocolate
- 3/4 of a cup of creamy almond butter
- 2 tablespoons of coconut oil
- 1/2 a cup of pureed prunes

Preparation:

- Take a large sized baking sheet and line it up with parchment paper
- Take a large sized bowl and add quinoa, oats, almonds, chia seeds, chocolate and cherries
- Take a small saucepan and place It over low heat
- Add almond butter, coconut oil, and 1/2 a teaspoon of salt
- Stir well until the whole mixture is smooth and has melted
- Pour the almond butter mix over the oat mix and stir well
- Use your hands to form bars and place them on your parchment paper

- Chill for 3 hours
- Enjoy!

Nutrition Values

- Calories: 286
- Fat: 17g
- Carbohydrates: 33g
- Protein: 8g

Grilled Up Asparagus

Prepping time: 15 minutes
Cooking time: 3 minutes
For 4 servings

Ingredients:

- 1 pound of fresh asparagus spears trimmed up
- 1 tablespoon of olive oil
- Salt as needed
- Pepper as needed

Preparation:

- Pre-heat your grill to high heat
- Coat the asparagus spears with olive oil
- Season with pepper and salt
- Grill for 2-3 minutes until tender
- Enjoy!

Nutrition Values

- Calories: 56
- Fat: 3.2g
- Carbohydrates: 4g
- Protein: 2g

Simply Delicious Crispy Potatoes and Cabbage

Prepping time: 25 minutes
Cooking time: 40 minutes
For 4 servings

Ingredients:

- 1/3 a cup of olive oil
- 5 thinly sliced carrots
- 1 thinly sliced onion
- 1 teaspoon of sea salt
- 1/2 a teaspoon of ground black pepper
- 1/2 a teaspoon of ground cumin
- 1/4 a teaspoon of ground turmeric
- 1/2 of a shredded cabbage head
- 5 peeled potatoes cut into 1-inch cubes

Preparation:

- Take a skillet and place it over medium heat then pour in olive oil
- Add carrots and the onion then cook them for 5 minutes
- Stir in salt, cumin, pepper, turmeric, cabbage and cook for 15-20 minutes
- Add potatoes
- Cover and lower down the heat to medium-low
- Cook for 20-30 minutes until the potatoes are tender

Nutrition Values

- Calories: 415
- Fat: 20g
- Carbohydrates: 52g
- Protein: 7g

Healthy Broccoli Bites

Prepping time: 10 minutes
Cooking time: 15 minutes
For 6 servings

Ingredients:

- 2 separate broccoli heads (florets)
- 2 teaspoons of extra virgin olive oil
- 1 teaspoon of sea salt
- 1/2 a teaspoon of ground black pepper
- 1 minced garlic clove
- 1 teaspoon of lemon juice

Preparation:

- Pre-heat your oven to 400 degrees Fahrenheit
- Take a large sized bowl and add broccoli florets alongside olive oil
- Add sea salt, garlic, and pepper then mix well
- Spread the broccoli in an even layer on a baking sheet
- Bake in your oven for 15-20 minutes (make sure to poke occasionally using a long fork)
- Remove once done and transfer them onto your serving platter
- Squeeze lemon juice and serve!

Nutrition Values

- Calories: 49
- Fat: 2g
- Carbohydrates: 0g
- Protein: 3g

Super Sweet Potato Sticks

Prepping time: 15 minutes
Cooking time: 40 minutes
For 4 servings

Ingredients:

- 1 tablespoon of olive oil
- 1/2 a teaspoon of paprika
- 8 pieces of sweet potatoes sliced up into lengthwise quarters

Preparation:

- Pre-heat your oven to 400 degrees Fahrenheit
- Take a baking sheet and spray it with vegetable oil
- Take a large sized bowl, add paprika and olive oil then mix them well
- Add the potato sticks and stir well to coat them
- Place them onto your prepared baking sheet
- Bake for 40 minutes in your oven
- Enjoy!

Nutrition Values

- Calories: 243
- Fat: 4g
- Carbohydrates: 52g
- Protein: 7g

Seasoned Sugar Snap Peas

Prepping time: 10 minutes
Cooking time: 8 minutes
For 4 servings

Ingredients:

- 1 pound of sugar snap peas
- 1 tablespoon of olive oil
- 1 tablespoon of chopped up shallots
- 1 teaspoon of chopped up fresh thymes
- Kosher salt

Preparation:

- Pre-heat your oven to 450 degrees Fahrenheit
- Take a medium sized baking sheet and spread the sugar snap peas in a single layer
- Lather them with olive oil
- Sprinkle thyme, shallot and kosher salt
- Bake for 6-8 minutes
- Enjoy!

Nutrition Values

- Calories: 59
- Fat: 4g
- Carbohydrates: 5g
- Protein: 1.4g

Local's Favorite Pad Thai

Prepping time: 5 minutes
Cooking time: 0 minutes
For 4 servings

Ingredients:

- 1 large sized zucchini
- 2 large to medium sized carrots
- 1 piece of capsicum
- 4 oyster mushrooms
- 1 cup of red cabbage
- 1/2 a cup of spring onions
- 1/4 a cup of sesame seeds
- 1/4 of a cup of peanut butter (for sauce)
- 3 tablespoons of tamari (for sauce)
- 4 tablespoons of water (for sauce)

Preparation:

- Spiralize the zucchini and carrots or thinly slice them (as preferred)
- Cut up the remaining vegetables
- Take a bowl and add the sauce ingredients
- Once done, add veggies and sauce together a bowl
- Garnish with some sesame seeds
- Enjoy!

Nutrition Values

- Calories: 563
- Fat: 45g
- Carbohydrates: 23g
- Protein: 20g

Hearty Black Beans and Quinoa

Prepping time: 15 minutes
Cooking time: 35 minutes
For 10 servings

Ingredients:

- 1 teaspoon of vegetable oil
- 1 chopped onion
- 2 chopped garlic cloves
- 3/4 cup of quinoa
- 1 cup of vegetable broth
- 1 teaspoon of ground cumin
- 1/4 teaspoon of cayenne pepper
- Salt as needed
- Ground black pepper
- 1 cup of frozen corn kernels
- 2 cans of black beans (drained and rinsed)
- 1/2 a cup of chopped up fresh cilantro

Preparation:

- Take a medium sized saucepan and place it over medium heat
- Add oil and heat it up
- Add the onion and garlic then cook for 10 minutes
- Next, add quinoa into the onion mixture and cover it with vegetable broth
- Season with cayenne pepper, cumin, salt, and pepper
- Bring the mix to a boil
- Cover it up and lower down the heat

- Simmer for 20 minutes until the quinoa is tender and the broth is finely absorbed
- Stir in the frozen corn into the saucepan and simmer for 5 minutes
- Add black beans into the cilantro and enjoy!

Nutrition Values

- Calories: 145
- Fat: 2.5g
- Carbohydrates: 12g
- Protein: 9g

Healthy Brussel Sprout Poppers

Prepping time: 15 minutes
Cooking time: 45 minutes
For 6 servings

Ingredients:

- 1 and a 1/2 pound of Brussels sprouts, make sure the ends are trimmed up and the yellow leaves removed
- 2 tablespoons of olive oil
- 1 teaspoon of kosher salt
- 1/2 a teaspoon of freshly ground black pepper

Preparation:

- Pre-heat your oven to 400 degrees Fahrenheit
- Add trimmed Brussels sprouts, kosher salt, olive oil, and pepper then place it into a large re-sealable bag
- Seal it up tightly and shake it around
- Transfer the contents onto a baking sheet
- Roast for 30-45 minutes, making sure to shake and mix everything around every 5-7 minutes
- Lower down the heat
- Once they are looking crisp and are almost black, take them out and season with some salt
- Serve and enjoy!

Nutrition Values

- Calories: 97
- Fat: 5g
- Carbohydrates: 9g
- Protein: 3g

Tasty Vegan Fried Rice

Prepping time: 5 minutes
Cooking time: 7 minutes
For 6 servings

Ingredients:

- 1 teaspoon of sesame oil
- 1 cup of chopped carrots
- 4 sliced scallions
- 2 minced garlic cloves
- 1/2 a teaspoon of chopped fresh ginger
- 1/2 a block of crumbled firm tofu
- 1/4 teaspoon of turmeric
- 1/2 a cup of edamame
- 4 cups of cooked brown rice
- 1-2 tablespoons of soy sauce
- Fresh cilantro

Preparation:

- Take a large skillet and place it over heat
- Add oil and heat it up
- Add scallions and carrots then sauté for 5 minutes
- Next, add garlic and ginger then sauté for an additional minute
- Toss crumbled tofu into the skillet alongside turmeric
- Add soy sauce and rice
- Mix it around and enjoy!

Nutrition Values

- Calories: 425
- Fat: 31g
- Carbohydrates: 2g
- Protein: 28g

Simple Coconut Rice

Prepping time: 5 minutes
Cooking time: 25 minutes
For 6 servings

Ingredients:

- 2 and a 1/2 cups of Basmati rice
- 5 cans of coconut milk
- 1 pinch of salt

Preparation:

- Take a large sized saucepan and place it over high heat
- Add in the rice, salt, and coconut milk
- Bring the mixture to a boil
- Lower down the heat and simmer for 25 minutes
- Enjoy!

Nutrition Values

- Calories: 545
- Fat:34g
- Carbohydrates: 52g
- Protein: 9g

Amazing Walnut Hummus – Perfect as a Veggie Dip!

Prepping time: 10 minutes
Cooking time: 6 minutes
For 2 servings

Ingredients:

- 500g of drained chickpeas
- 2 cloves of garlic
- 1 large roasted pepper
- 1 tablespoon of tahini paste
- Juice from 1/2 of a lemon
- 4 chopped up walnut halves
- 2 pieces of courgettes cut up into batons
- 2 pieces of carrots cut up into batons
- 2 pieces of celery sticks cut up into batons

Preparation:

- Take a small sized bowl and add in the chickpeas, garlic, lemon juice and pepper
- Blitz the mixture in a food processor until you have a nice and thick puree
- Stir in the walnuts
- Serve with your favorite veggies!

Nutrition Values

- Protein: 14g
- Carbs: 30g
- Fats: 15g
- Calories: 296

Summer Squash Special

Prepping time: 15 minutes
Cooking time: 30 minutes
For 4 servings

Ingredients:

- 1 tablespoon of vegetable oil
- 1 small sized sliced onion
- 2 medium sized chopped up tomatoes
- 1 teaspoon of salt
- 1/4 teaspoon of pepper
- 2 small zucchinis cut up into 1/2-inch slices
- 1 bay leaf
- 1/2 a teaspoon of dried basil

Preparation:

- Take a large sized skillet and place it over medium heat
- Heat up some oil
- Stir in onions and cook for 5 minutes
- Add tomatoes and season with some salt and pepper
- Keep stirring and cooking for 5 minutes
- Add zucchini, the bay leaf, yellow squash, and basil
- Cover it up and bring the heat down to low
- Simmer for 20 minutes
- Remove the bay leaf and serve!

Nutrition Values

- Calories: 70
- Fat: 5g
- Carbohydrates: 5g
- Protein: 2g

Healthy Mushrooms and White Wine

Prepping time: 15 minutes
Cooking time: 30 minutes
For 6 servings

Ingredients:

- 1 tablespoon of olive oil
- 1 pound of fresh mushrooms
- 1 teaspoon of Italian seasoning
- 1/4 cup of dry white wine
- 2 minced cloves of garlic
- Salt as needed
- Pepper as needed
- 2 tablespoons of chopped up fresh chives

Preparation:

- Take a skillet and place it over medium heat
- Heat up the oil
- Add mushrooms alongside Italian seasoning and cook for about 10 minutes
- Add wine and garlic to the skillet
- Keep cooking until the wine has evaporated
- Season with pepper and salt
- Sprinkle chives and cook for 1 more minute
- Enjoy!

Nutrition Values

- Calories: 60
- Fat: 3g
- Carbohydrates: 5.6g
- Protein: 13g

Trendy Mexican Rice

Prepping time: 20 minutes
Cooking time: 30 minutes
For 8 servings

Ingredients:

- 2 tablespoons of vegetable oil
- 2/3 cup of diced onion
- 1 cup of uncooked rice
- 1 cup of chopped green bell pepper
- 1 teaspoon of ground cumin
- 1 teaspoon of chili powder
- 1 can of tomato sauce
- 2 teaspoons of salt
- 1 minced garlic clove
- 3 cups of water

Preparation:

- Take a large sized saucepan and add vegetable oil over medium-low heat
- Allow it to heat up then add the onion and sauté until golden
- Add rice to the pan and stir well to coat the grains with oil
- Add the green bell pepper, chili powder, cumin, tomato sauce, garlic, salt, and water
- Cover and bring to a boil
- Lower down the heat and allow it to simmer for 30-40 minutes
- Stir well
- Enjoy!

Nutrition Values

- Calories: 187
- Fat: 5g
- Carbohydrates: 33g
- Protein: 4g

Fancy Fried Onions

Prepping time: 15 minutes
Cooking time: 20 minutes
For 12 servings

Ingredients:

- 1 quart of vegetable oil
- 1 cup of all-purpose flour
- 1 cup of beer (can also be replaced with water)
- 1 pinch of salt
- 1 pinch of ground black pepper
- 4 pieces of onions peeled and sliced up into rings

Preparation:

- Take a large sized deep skillet and heat up the oil at 365 degrees Fahrenheit
- Mix the flour, beer, flour, pepper and salt
- Drench the onions in the mix until they are coated well
- Deep fry the onions until they are golden brown
- Drain and enjoy

Nutrition Values

- Calories: 135
- Fat: 8g
- Carbohydrates: 12g
- Protein: 1g

Mini Baked Tofu Bites

Prepping time: 10 minutes
Cooking time: 15 minutes
For 4 servings

Ingredients:

- 1 pack of extra firm tofu
- 1/3 cup of soy sauce
- 1 tablespoon of maple syrup
- 1 tablespoon of ketchup
- 1 tablespoon of vinegar
- 1 tablespoon of sesame seeds
- 1/4 teaspoon of garlic powder
- 1/4 teaspoon of ground black pepper

Preparation:

- Pre-heat your oven to 375 degrees Fahrenheit
- Take a nonstick baking sheet and spray with oil
- Slice up the tofu into 1/2-inch slices and gently remove the excess water out of the tofu
- Cut the tofu into 1/2-inch cubes
- Take a bowl and stir in soy sauce, ketchup, maple syrup, and vinegar
- Stir in sesame seeds, black pepper, and garlic powder
- Gently stir the tofu into the sauce
- Cover up and marinate for 5 minutes
- Add tofu into the baking sheet in a single layer
- Bake in your pre-heated oven for 15 minutes
- Turn the tofu and bake until a golden-brown texture shows (usually takes around 15 minutes)

- Enjoy!

Nutrition Values

- Calories: 175
- Fat: 9g
- Carbohydrates: 14g
- Protein: 12g

Ancient Japanese Sesame Beans

Prepping time: 5 minutes
Cooking time: 15 minutes
For 4 servings

Ingredients:

- 1 tablespoon of canola oil
- 1 clove of minced garlic
- 1 teaspoon of sesame oil
- 1 pound of fresh green beans
- 1 tablespoon of soy sauce
- 2 tablespoons of toasted sesame seeds

Preparation:

- Take a large sized skillet and place it over medium heat
- Once the skillet is hot add in the canola and sesame oil
- Add the green beans and garlic and stir well until they are fully coated
- Cook until the beans are bright green and show slightly brown spots, should take around 10 minutes
- Remove the heat and stir in soy sauce
- Cover for 5 minutes
- Transfer to a serving platter and sprinkle some toasted sesame seeds
- Enjoy!

Nutrition Values

- Calories: 100
- Fat: 6g
- Carbohydrates: 10g
- Protein: 3g

Simple Sweet Pepper Skillet

Prepping time: 15 minutes
Cooking time: 10 minutes
For 4 servings

Ingredients:

- 1 teaspoon of extra virgin olive oil
- 1 teaspoon of sesame oil
- 4 thinly sliced green bell peppers
- 1 chopped up yellow bell pepper
- 1 chopped up red bell peppers
- 1 chopped up red onion
- 2 teaspoons of minced garlic
- 1/4 teaspoon of salt
- 1/4 teaspoon of ground black pepper

Preparation:

- Take a large sized skillet and place it over medium heat
- Add olive oil and sesame oil, allow them to heat up
- Add the peppers, red onion, garlic, pepper, and salt
- Cook and stir for about 7-10 minutes until the peppers are cooked thoroughly
- Enjoy!

Nutrition Values

- Calories: 90
- Fat: 4g
- Carbohydrates: 10g
- Protein: 3g

Mini Hummus Pizza Bites

Prepping time: 15 minutes
Cooking time: 10 minutes
For 4 servings

Ingredients:

- 2 tablespoons of hummus
- 1 naan bread
- 1 and 1/2 cups of arugula
- 1 pitted and finely chopped date
- 2 teaspoons of pumpkin seeds
- 1 teaspoon of balsamic vinegar

Preparation:

- Spread the hummus on top of the Naan bread
- Top it up with arugula, pumpkin seeds and date
- Drizzle vinegar over the pizza
- Enjoy!

Nutrition Values

- Calories: 360
- Fat: 9g
- Carbohydrates: 56g
- Protein: 16g

Chapter 5
Dessert Recipes

Fluffy Tofu Cake

Prepping time: 10 minutes
Cooking time: 20 minutes
For 8 servings

Ingredients:

- 2 packs of extra firm drained and cubed tofu
- 1 cup of white sugar
- 1 teaspoon of vanilla extract
- 1/4 teaspoon of salt
- 1/4 cup of vegetable oil
- 2 and 1/2 tablespoons of lemon juice
- 1 (9 inch) sized prepared graham cracker crust

Preparation:

- Pre-heat your oven to 350 degrees Fahrenheit
- Take a blender or food processor and add sugar, tofu, vanilla, salt, vegetable oil, and lemon juice
- Blend the whole mixture well
- Pour the mixture into your prepared crust
- Bake in your oven for 20-30 minutes
- Remove it from the oven and allow it to cool
- Refrigerate until it is chilled
- Enjoy!

Nutrition Values

- Calories: 365
- Fat: 15g
- Carbohydrates: 42g
- Protein: 12g

Icy Fruit Salad

Prepping time: 15 minutes
Cooking time: 0 minutes
For 6 servings

Ingredients:

- 1/3 a cup of white sugar
- 2 cups of water
- 1 can of frozen orange juice concentrate, thawed
- 1 can of frozen lemonade concentrated, thawed
- 5 sliced bananas
- 20 ounces can of crushed pineapple with juice
- 2 packs of frozen strawberries thawed

Preparation:

- Dissolve the sugar in water
- Add orange juice, bananas, lemonade, crushed pineapple, and juice
- Pour the mixture into a 9x13 glass pan
- Freeze until it is solid
- Allow it to sit for 5 minutes and cut it out
- Serve and enjoy!

Nutrition Values

- Calories: 325
- Fat: 1g
- Carbohydrates: 68g
- Protein: 3g

Chocolate Chunk Tofu Pudding

Prepping time: 10 minutes
Cooking time: 0 minutes
For 6 servings

Ingredients:

- 1 banana broken up into chunks
- 1 pack of soft silken tofu
- 1/4 cup of powdered sugar
- 5 tablespoons of unsweetened cocoa powder
- 3 tablespoons of soy milk
- 1 pinch of ground cinnamon

Preparation:

- Take a blender and add banana, sugar, tofu, cocoa powder, cinnamon and soy milk
- Mix everything well and blend
- Puree until it is nice and smooth
- Pour the mixture into serving dishes
- Allow it to chill for an hour and serve!

Nutrition Values

- Calories: 134
- Fat: 5g
- Carbohydrates: 18g
- Protein: 6g

Extravagant Basil Lime Sorbet

Prepping time: 30 minutes
Cooking time: 50 minutes
For 6 servings

Ingredients:

- 1 cup of sugar
- 1 cup of water
- 3/4 cup of fresh lime juice
- 15 pieces of fresh basil minced up

Preparation:

- Make the syrup by taking a saucepan and placing it over medium heat
- Add the sugar and water then bring it to a boil for 1 minute
- Remove the heat
- Add the syrup, basil and lime juice in a blender
- Puree the whole mixture well and pour it to another container
- Store in your freezer and allow it to cool for 2 hours
- Break the frozen mix into pieces and add them to your blender
- Blend again until it is smooth
- Return it to the container and allow it to chill
- Serve and enjoy!

Nutrition Values

- Calories: 95
- Fat: 2g
- Carbohydrates: 25g
- Protein: 1g

Classic Vegan Chocolate Pie

Prepping time: 15 minutes
Cooking time: 25 minutes
For 8 servings

Ingredients:

- 1 pound of silken tofu
- 1 cup of unsweetened cocoa powder
- 1 cup of white sugar
- 1 tablespoon of vanilla extract
- 1/2 a teaspoon of cider vinegar
- 1 prepared gram cracker crust

Preparation:

- Pre-heat your oven to 375 degrees Fahrenheit
- Take an electric mixer and add tofu then blend until smooth
- Add in cocoa, vanilla, sugar, vinegar then blend well until a smooth mixture forms
- Pour the mixture into your crust
- Bake in your oven for 25 minutes
- Allow it to chill for 1 hour and serve!

Nutrition Values

- Calories: 280
- Fat: 10g
- Carbohydrates: 44g
- Protein: 6g

Healthy Banana Cookie Bites

Prepping time: 15 minutes
Cooking time: 20 minutes
For 36 servings

Ingredients:

- 4 ripe bananas
- 2 cups of rolled oats
- 1 cup of pitted and chopped dates
- 2 cups of vegetable oil
- 1 teaspoon of vanilla extract

Preparation:

- Pre-heat your oven to 350 degrees Fahrenheit
- Take a large sized bowl and mash up the bananas
- Stir in the oats, oil, dates, vanilla into the mashed bananas and allow the mixture to rest for 15 minutes
- Scoop up the mixture using a teaspoon and place the spoonful's onto an ungreased cookie sheet
- Bake for 20 minutes in your pre-heated oven until it is lightly brown
- Enjoy!

Nutrition Values

- Calories: 60
- Fat: 2g
- Carbohydrates: 9g
- Protein: 1g

Simple Strawberry Medley

Prepping time: 10 minutes
Cooking time: 0 minutes
For 6 servings

Ingredients:

- 16 ounces of fresh strawberries with the large berries cut in half
- 1 tablespoon of balsamic vinegar
- 1/3 cup of white sugar

Preparation:

- Take a bowl and add in the strawberries
- Drizzle vinegar over the strawberries and sprinkle sugar
- Stir gently and allow it to combine together
- Cover it up and let it sit for 1-4 hours
- Enjoy!

Nutrition Values

- Calories: 60
- Fat: 0.2g
- Carbohydrates: 14g
- Protein: 0.5g

Spongy Vegan Cake

Prepping time: 15 minutes
Cooking time: 30 minutes
For 16 servings

Ingredients:

- 1 large peeled orange
- 1 and 1/2 cups of all-purpose flour
- 1 cup of white sugar
- 1/3 a cup of vegetable oil
- 1 teaspoon of baking soda
- 1/4 teaspoon of salt

Preparation:

- Pre-heat your oven to 375 degrees Fahrenheit
- Take an 8x8 inch baking pan and grease it up
- Grab a blender and blend the orange until liquefied
- Measure 1 cup of orange juice
- Whisk in orange juice, vegetable oil, flour, sugar, baking soda, and salt into a bowl
- Mix well
- Pour the prepared batter into your prepped pan
- Bake in the oven for 30 minutes or until you are able to put a toothpick in the cake and it comes out clean.
- Enjoy!

Nutrition Values

- Calories: 145
- Fat: 7g
- Carbohydrates: 19g
- Protein: 2g

Oatmeal Chia Seed Cookies

Prepping time: 15 minutes
Cooking time: 10 minutes
For 12 servings

Ingredients:

- 2 cups of rolled oats
- 1 cup of brown sugar
- 2/3 cup of whole wheat flour
- 3 tablespoons of chia seeds
- 1 teaspoon of ground cinnamon
- 1 teaspoon of baking soda
- 1/2 a teaspoon of baking powder
- 1/2 a teaspoon of salt
- 2/3 cup of applesauce (unsweetened works well)
- 3 tablespoon of coconut oil
- 1 cup of dried cranberries
- 1/4 cup of shredded unsweetened coconut

Preparation:

- Pre-heat your oven to 350 degrees Fahrenheit
- Take a baking sheet and line it up with parchment paper
- Grab a bowl and add in brown sugar, oats, cinnamon, flour, chia seeds, baking soda, salt, and baking powder
- Mix well
- Stir in applesauce, coconut oil, and oat mix then mix until the dough is evenly prepared
- Toss in cranberries and coconut into the dough and mix well
- Spoon the dough onto your baking sheet

- Bake for 10-15 minutes make sure the cookies are lightly browned up
- Enjoy!

Nutrition Values

- Calories: 280
- Fat: 8g
- Carbohydrates: 37g
- Protein: 3g

Almond Dashed Vanilla Cocoroons

Prepping time: 15 minutes
Cooking time: 20 minutes
For 15 servings

Ingredients:

- 2 cups of unsweetened coconut milk
- 3/4 cup of almond flour
- 7 tablespoons of maple syrup
- 4 tablespoons of coconut oil
- 1 tablespoon of vanilla extract
- 1 teaspoon of almond extract
- 1/4 teaspoon of sea salt

Preparation:

- Pre-heat your oven to 200 degrees Fahrenheit
- Line a baking sheet with parchment paper
- Add the coconut, maple syrup, almond flour, vanilla extract, coconut oil, almond extract, and salt into your food processor
- Blend well, making sure to scrape down the sides if needed
- Scoop the mixture using cookie scoops and form mounds on your baking sheet
- Bake in your oven for 20 minutes
- Turn the heat off
- Keep the cookies in the oven until they are cooled and dried out, should take around 3-8 hours
- Enjoy!

Nutrition Values

- Calories: 125
- Fat: 10g
- Carbohydrates: 11g
- Protein: 1.5g

Sweet Melon Almond Salad with Watercress

Prepping time: 15 minutes
Cooking time: 0 minutes
For 4 servings

Ingredients:

- 3 tablespoons of fresh lime juice
- 1 teaspoon of white sugar
- 1 teaspoon of minced fresh ginger
- 1/4 cup of vegetable oil
- 2 bunches of trimmed and chopped watercress
- 3 cups of cubed watermelon
- 2 cups of cubed cantaloupe
- 1/3 cup of toasted and sliced almonds

Preparation:

- Take a large sized bowl and whisk in lime juice, ginger and sugar
- Gradually add oil and season with some pepper and salt
- Add watercress, cantaloupe, watermelon to the dressing mixture and toss well
- Transfer to a salad plate and serve with sprinkles of sliced almond
- Serve and enjoy!

Nutrition Values

- Calories: 250
- Fat: 14g
- Carbohydrates: 21g
- Protein: 7g

Amazing Vegan Banana Ice Cream

Prepping time: 10 minutes
Cooking time: 0 minutes
For 2 servings

Ingredients:

- 2 large sized frozen bananas cut up into small chunks
- 1 cup of unsweetened almond milk
- 1 tablespoon of chopped pecans
- 1 pinch of ground cinnamon
- 1/2 cup of chopped up dark chocolate

Preparation:

- Blend bananas, pecans, almond milk, cinnamon in a food processor
- Mix well until it is smooth and creamy
- Chill and serve with dark chocolate sprinkled on top

Nutrition Values

- Calories: 180
- Fat: 4g
- Carbohydrates: 32g
- Protein: 2g

Quick and Delicious Berry Pops

Prepping time: 15 minutes
Cooking time: 0 minutes
For 12 servings

Ingredients:

- 16 ounces of blueberries
- 16 ounces of hulled strawberries
- 16 ounces of raspberries
- 1/2 a cup of brown sugar
- 2 and a 1/2 cups of vanilla soy milk

Preparation:

- Add blueberries, strawberries, and raspberries into your blender (in batches) and blend them
- Strain the mixture into a medium sized bowl
- Pour brown sugar onto the berries
- Stir in soy milk until it is blended well
- Pour mixture into small paper cups, making sure to fill them up to about 2/3rds
- Make sure to insert a holding stick and freeze for about 2-3 hours
- Enjoy!

Nutrition Values

- Calories: 90
- Fat: 1g
- Carbohydrates: 15g
- Protein: 1.8g

Sugary Snow Cone Delight

Prepping time: 5 minutes
Cooking time: 0 minutes
For 2 servings

Ingredients:

- 1 and a 1/2 cup of shaved ice
- 3/4 can of cola flavored carbonated beverage

Preparation:

- Take a medium sized bowl and stir together the snow and your desired cola
- Serve immediately and enjoy with some vegan whipped cream topping if needed!

Nutrition Values

- Calories: 75
- Fat: 2g
- Carbohydrates: 14g
- Protein: 0g

Sweet Apple Kale Soup

Prepping time: 20 minutes
Cooking time: 15 minutes
For 2 servings

Ingredients:

- 8 walnut halves broken up into pieces
- 1 finely chopped up onion
- 2 coarsely grated carrots
- 2 unpeeled but finely chopped up red apples
- 1 tablespoon of cider vinegar
- 500ml of reduced salt vegetable stock
- 200g of roughly chopped kale
- 20g of dried apple crisps

Preparation:

- Take a non-stick frying pan or skillet and add walnuts, stir fry them for about 3 minutes until they are toasty
- Remove the heat and let the mixture cool
- Take a large sized saucepan and add carrots, vinegar, onion, and apples then bring the mix to a boil
- Bring the heat down to low and simmer for about 10 minutes, making sure to keep stirring the mixture
- Wait till the apples are tender and simmer for another 2 minutes
- Transfer the mix to a blender and blend the mix until it is smooth
- Pour the soup into your serving bowl and garnish with a bit of toasted walnuts
- Serve!

Nutrition Values

- Protein: 12g
- Carbs: 26g
- Fats: 21g
- Calories: 403

Ginger Mango Sorbet

Prepping time: 10 minutes
Cooking time: 10 minutes
For 8 servings

Ingredients:

- 1 and a 1/2 cup of water
- 2 cups of white sugar
- 1 piece of fresh ginger peeled and sliced up
- 1 pinch of sea salt
- 1 teaspoon of lime zest
- 2 cups of orange juice
- 1 cup of mango juice
- 1/3 cup of lemon juice

Preparation:

- Take a saucepan and add water, ginger, sugar, salt, and lime zest
- Bring the mixture to a boil
- Bring the heat down to low and allow it to simmer for 5 minutes
- Allow the mixture to cool
- Stir in orange juice, lemon juice and mango juice
- Cover and chill for about 3 hours
- Cut it up into cubes and add the ice to the blender and mix
- Enjoy!

Nutrition Values

- Calories: 185
- Fat: 0.5g
- Carbohydrates: 49g
- Protein: 1g

Sugar Date Nut Bars

Prepping time: 15 minutes
Cooking time: 45 minutes
For 16 servings

Ingredients:

- 2/3 cup of unbleached all-purpose flour
- 2/3 cup of packed brown sugar
- 1/2 cup of finely chopped walnuts
- 1 teaspoon of ground cinnamon
- 1/4 teaspoon of ground cardamom
- 1/4 teaspoon of salt
- 1/2 a teaspoon of baking powder
- 1 cup of pitted and chopped dates

Preparation:

- Pre-heat your oven to 350 degrees Fahrenheit
- Lightly oil up an 8-inch square baking pan
- Take a large bowl and add flour, brown sugar, walnuts, cardamom, cinnamon, baking powder, salt, and dates
- Mix and beat the mixture well
- Spoon the batter into your pan and bake in your oven for 25 minutes

Nutrition Values

- Calories: 120
- Fat: 3g
- Carbohydrates: 25g
- Protein: 1.8g

Icy Watermelon Blend with Champagne

Prepping time: 15 minutes
Cooking time: 0 minutes
For 16 servings

Ingredients:

- 2 pounds of cubed watermelon
- 1/2 a cup of white sugar
- 1 cup of champagne (can also be replaced with water)
- 4 slices of watermelon

Preparation:

- Add cubed watermelon and sugar to a blender and blend everything for 1 minute
- Stir in champagne and pour the mixture into a plastic container
- Cover and freeze for 2 hours making sure to stir after every 30 minutes
- Serve by removing the frozen mix from the freezer and stirring it well using a fork
- Serve in tall glasses with sliced up watermelons on the side
- Enjoy!

Nutrition Values

- Calories: 245
- Fat: 1g
- Carbohydrates: 55g
- Protein: 3.2g

Classic Candy Apples

Prepping time: 5 minutes
Cooking time: 20 minutes
For 8 servings

Ingredients:

- 8 whole apples
- 3 cups of white sugar
- 1/2 a cup of white corn syrup
- 1/2 a cup of water
- 8 cinnamon candies
- 1 teaspoon of red food coloring

Preparation:

- Insert a wood craft stick into the bottom of your apples
- Take a baking sheet and grease it well
- Next, take a heavy saucepan and add sugar, corn syrup, and water then place it over medium heat
- Keep heating it until the temperature reaches 270-290 degrees Fahrenheit without stirring it
- Remove the heat once the desired temperature is reached and stir in the candy and food coloring
- Hold the apples by the stick and twirl them in the prepared syrup, making sure to tilt the pan until they are full covered
- Place them on your baking sheet and allow them to cool
- Enjoy!

Nutrition Values

- Calories: 420
- Fat: 2g
- Carbohydrates: 75g
- Protein: 1g

Delicious Vegan Gelatin Treat

Prepping time: 10 minutes
Cooking time: 0 minutes
For 12 servings

Ingredients:

- 1/2 a teaspoon of cornstarch
- 2 teaspoons of water
- 2 cups of cherry juice
- 1 teaspoon of agar-agar

Preparation:

- Take a small cup and mix the cornstarch with water
- Keep it on the side
- Take a saucepan and add 1 and a 1/2 cup of cheery juice, and all of the agar-agar powder
- Allow it to stand for 5 minutes until it is soft
- Place it over medium high heat and allow it to simmer for just 1 minute
- Remove the heat and stir in the rest of the juice alongside the cornstarch mix and mix well
- Pour the mix into small serving cups and allow it to chill for 4 hours
- Serve!

Nutrition Values

- Calories: 30
- Fat: 1g
- Carbohydrates: 6g
- Protein: 2g

Conclusion

I really want to thank you for reading this book. I sincerely hope you received value from it!

Like I said, these are my favorite recipes that have helped me change my life and body. I followed what I put in this book, and I was able to lose weight and gain muscle. If you apply this knowledge towards your own life then I have no doubt you can start to see a positive change in your soul, mind, and body!

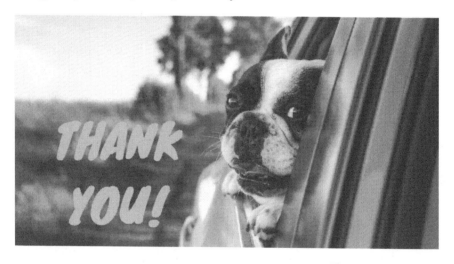

If you received value from this book, then I'd like to ask you for a favor. Would you be kind enough to leave a review for this book on Amazon?

<u>Click Here to Leave a Review on Amazon!</u>
https://www.amazon.com/review/create-review/ref=dpx_acr_wr_link?asin=B076YZZKMV#

I want to help as many people as I can with this book; more reviews will help me to accomplish that!

Free Beginner's Guide to Plant-Based Fitness!

Take your knowledge to the next level. Expand on what you learned and start to take action. In this free guide, you will learn more recipes for a breakfast, lunch, dinner, and for snacking, what a vegan day may look like, and how to fix common mistakes at the gym. You will also be getting a free workout routine template to help you get started!

Click Here to Get Your Free Guide!

Preview:

One of the biggest sources of frustration many vegans and vegetarians have when it comes to their fitness and health is what in the world to do at the gym. Many instructors out there don't understand the intricacies of a plant-based diet; so, their routines and programs are centered around heavy gains with lots of meat eating- yuck! Luckily for you, Buff Veggie is here to help you along your way!

A change you can make right away to how you approach working out is how much time you spend at the gym. Most of us correlate time spent at the gym with how much muscle we will gain- however this is simply not the case. The recommended time one should spend working out with weights (not cardio) is no more than 45 minutes. After that, your body is too exhausted and "beat up" to repair fully. Spending more time at the gym does not equal more results- focus on the fundamentals of your workouts and the results will come.

Continue reading in the free guide! Get It *Here*

http://bit.ly/2vy3zFs

Go to Buffveggie.com for helpful guides on how to make these delicious recipes!

Learn about mistakes you need to correct in the gym, the best supplements to take, how becoming vegan can help your heart, and much, much more! Enjoy multiple articles each week that are aimed at getting you in the best possible shape while remaining 100% plant-based!

Check Out the Blog Here http://buffveggie.com/

Once again, thank you so much for reading this book! Good luck in all your future endeavors!

Printed in Great Britain
by Amazon